T0134824

Cancer Drug Discovery and Development

Series Editor
Beverly A. Teicher
Bethesda, Maryland, USA

Cancer Drug Discovery and Development, the Springer series headed by Beverly A. Teicher, is the definitive book series in cancer research and oncology. Volumes cover the process of drug discovery, preclinical models in cancer research, specific drug target groups, and experimental and approved therapeutic agents. The volumes are current and timely, anticipating areas where experimental agents are reaching FDA approval. Each volume is edited by an expert in the field covered, and chapters are authored by renowned scientists and physicians in their fields of interest.

More information about this series at http://www.springer.com/series/7625

Yuzhuo Wang • Francesco Crea
Editors

Tumor Dormancy and Recurrence

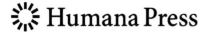 Humana Press

Editors
Yuzhuo Wang
Department of Experimental Therapeutics
and Department of Urologic Sciences
BC Cancer Agency and University of
British Columbia
Vancouver, BC, Canada

Francesco Crea
School of Life, Health & Chemical Sciences
The Open University, Walton Hall
Milton Keynes
Buckinghamshire, United Kingdom

ISSN 2196-9906 ISSN 2196-9914 (electronic)
Cancer Drug Discovery and Development
ISBN 978-3-319-86578-2 ISBN 978-3-319-59242-8 (eBook)
DOI 10.1007/978-3-319-59242-8

Printed on acid-free paper

This Humana Press imprint is published by Springer Nature
The registered company is Springer International Publishing AG
The registered company address is: Gewerbestrasse 11, 6330 Cham, Switzerland

Preface

Then Sleep and Death,
two twins of winged race,
of matchless swiftness,
but of silent pace

Homer, *The Iliad*, Book XVI. Pope's translation.

For several decades, cancer has been considered as a disease primarily characterized by unlimited and uncontrollable proliferation. Countless studies have drawn parallels between embryo and cancer cell growth [1], and cancer's "limitless replicative potential" is a milestone of the hallmarks paradigm [2].

In parallel with this view, a more nuanced description of cancer has gradually emerged. Laboratory experiments have shown that cancer cells are able not only to proliferate but also to alternate periods of quiescence with periods of rapid growth [3]. This reversible quiescent state is called "tumor dormancy" (from Latin *dormeo*: "I sleep"). In keeping with this paradigm, clinical observations have indicated that most neoplasms cannot be described in terms of unstoppable proliferation. For example, prostate cancer is characterized by prolonged iterative cycles of proliferation and dormancy (Fig. 1). Notably, during these periods of quiescence the neoplasm is often clinically indolent and therefore both patients and clinicians are less concerned about it.

The discovery of cancer dormancy paves the way for many unresolved questions. First of all: is cellular dormancy an inherited or acquired ability? How are cancer cells able to alternate proliferation and quiescence? And finally: why does tumor dormancy seem to be so critical for cancer cells' survival? Emerging evidence indicates that the mysterious phenomenon of cancer dormancy might hide the key for understanding the two deadliest attributes of cancer cells: their ability to resist anticancer treatments and their propensity to colonize distant organs. In the first two chapters of this book, Aguirre-Ghiso and Wang analyze the role of epigenetics and metabolic pathways in shaping the metastatic and drug-resistant potential of dormant cells.

Since dormant cells are generally overlooked by clinicians and resistant to conventional therapies, the "dormancy paradigm" paves the way for the development of

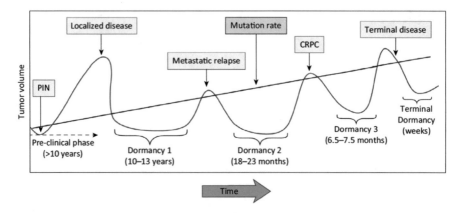

Fig. 1 The clinical course of prostate cancer is characterized by progressively shorter cycles of treatment– dormancy–relapse. The duration of the dormancy period is based on clinical evidence of progression-free survival after prostatectomy (1), androgen-deprivation therapy (2), and docetaxel treatment (3). An increased mutation rate (red line) correlates with shorter dormancy periods

a completely new class of therapies. In chapters "Tumor Dormancy, Angiogenesis and Metronomic Chemotherapy" and "Immunoncology of Dormant Tumors" of this book, Bocci and Bishop discuss the possible role of anti-angiogenic therapy and immunotherapy in targeting dormant cancer cells.

Finally, we decided to examine the roots of cancer dormancy by investigating the relationship between cancer proliferation, quiescence, and a thermodynamic description of biological processes (see chapter "Thermodynamics and Cancer Dormancy: A Perspective" by Tuszynski and Rietman). We hope that this chapter will identify new avenues of investigation for this fascinating research field.

We believe that this book is extremely timely and useful to everyone (students, clinicians, and scientists) who wants to understand more about the increasingly important concept cancer dormancy and recurrence. To produce an excellent text, we have decided to invite only outstanding contributors, with a strong track record of research in their specific area, and we have identified five key themes, corresponding to the chapters of this book. We hope that this first organic collection of essays on this topic will help to highlight the importance of this novel perspective, which has the potential to revolutionize our understanding of cancers and to pave the way for a new generation of therapies.

Vancouver, BC, Canada   Yuzhuo Wang
Walton Hall, Milton Keynes, UK   Francesco Crea

References

1. Monk M, Holding C (2001) Human embryonic genes re-expressed in cancer cells. Oncogene 20(56):8085–8091
2. Hanahan D, Weinberg RA (2011) Hallmarks of cancer: the next generation. Cell 144(5):646–674
3. Crea F, Nur Saidy NR, Collins CC, Wang Y (2015) The epigenetic/noncoding origin of tumor dormancy. Trends Mol Med. 21(4):206–211

Contents

Epigenetic Regulation of Cancer Dormancy as a Plasticity Mechanism for Metastasis Initiation

Maria Soledad Sosa, Emily Bernstein, and Julio A. Aguirre-Ghiso

Abstract Metastasis is responsible for the vast majority of cancer-related deaths. However, our understanding of this complex process is still vastly limited, as is the ability to prevent metastasis. Paradoxically, while clinical trials are commonly performed in patients with advanced metastatic disease, disseminated residual disease is rarely targeted. This eliminates a critical window of opportunity to prevent metastasis. Disseminated tumor cells (DTCs) that seed metastases can remain undetected years to decades after treatment of the primary tumor. Late relapse may be due to the ability of DTCs to survive in a quiescent or dormant state and evade therapies. Quiescence, a reversible growth arrest coupled to robust survival, has emerged as a fitting biological definition for dormancy of single DTCs, but these mechanisms

M.S. Sosa (✉)
Department of Pharmacological Sciences, Laboratory of Cancer Metastasis, Mount Sinai School of Medicine, New York, NY 10029, USA

Tisch Cancer Institute, Black Family Stem Cell Institute, Mount Sinai School of Medicine, New York, NY 10029, USA
e-mail: soledad.sosa@mssm.edu

E. Bernstein (✉)
Tisch Cancer Institute, Black Family Stem Cell Institute, Mount Sinai School of Medicine, New York, NY 10029, USA

Department of Oncological Sciences, Mount Sinai School of Medicine, New York, NY 10029, USA
e-mail: emily.bernstein@mssm.edu

J.A. Aguirre-Ghiso (✉)
Division of Hematology and Oncology, Department of Medicine, Mount Sinai School of Medicine, New York, NY 10029, USA

Department of Otolaryngology, Mount Sinai School of Medicine, New York, NY 10029, USA

Tisch Cancer Institute, Black Family Stem Cell Institute, Mount Sinai School of Medicine, New York, NY 10029, USA

Department of Oncological Sciences, Mount Sinai School of Medicine, New York, NY 10029, USA
e-mail: julio.aguirre-ghiso@mssm.edu

© Springer International Publishing AG 2017
Y. Wang, F. Crea (eds.), *Tumor Dormancy and Recurrence*, Cancer Drug Discovery and Development, DOI 10.1007/978-3-319-59242-8_1

remain as one of the least understood "black boxes" in cancer biology. Because of the reversible nature of dormancy, it has been proposed that epigenetic changes are key in regulating the onset, maintenance and reactivation from this state. This is mediated by the post-translational modification of histones (PTMs), ATP-dependent chromatin remodeling, DNA methylation, and the incorporation of specialized histone variants into chromatin. Many morphogenetic and micro-environmental cues like retinoic acid, TGFβs, hematopoietic stem cell dormancy regulating cues and BMPs are known to cause chromatin modifications that dictate cell fate; these same cues were linked to the induction of cancer cell dormancy. Despite progress in understanding cancer cell dormancy, key questions remain open regarding its epigenetic nature. In this chapter we attempt to address key questions related to this topic using available data or hypothetical scenarios to build a model to further dissect how cancer cell dormancy can be manipulated epigenetically as a therapeutic strategy.

Keywords Dormancy • Diapause • Dauer • Epigenome • Chromatin • Niche • Microenvironment • Metastasis • Relapse • Drug resistance • Differentiation • Senescence • MRD

Introduction

Metastasis is responsible for the vast majority of cancer-related deaths. However, our understanding of this complex process is still vastly limited, as is the ability to prevent metastatic development [1]. Paradoxically, clinical trials are commonly performed in patients with advanced metastatic disease, while therapies and approaches are commonly designed around the biology of primary tumors. Additionally, a fundamental problem is that disseminated residual disease is rarely targeted therapeutically and thus, a critical window of opportunity is missed to prevent metastasis [2, 3].

Metastases originate from **d**isseminated **t**umor **c**ells (DTCs), but it takes months to decades after treatment of the primary tumor for these lesions to develop [1]. It is clear that preventing late relapse is a major clinical need. For example, in breast cancer, >60% of all metastatic relapses occur beyond the 5 year mark post-treatment, a time during which patients are not commonly treated [4]. This scenario is also true for other solid cancers, including melanoma and head and neck cancers [1, 5, 6]. Clinical evidence suggests that improved outcomes within the first 5 years are due to advances in early detection, surgery and anti-proliferative therapies. This success has led to patients living longer. Nevertheless, they can still succumb to the cancer due to late recurrences. While a number of mechanisms may contribute, growing evidence suggests that late relapse may be due to the ability of DTCs to survive in a quiescent or dormant state and evade therapies [1, 7]. Quiescence, a reversible growth arrest coupled to robust survival, has emerged as a fitting biological definition for dormancy of single DTCs [1, 8]. Despite important advances in the modeling and understanding of cancer dormancy, this remains one of the least understood "black boxes" in cancer biology.

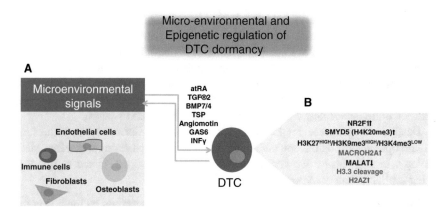

Fig. 1 (**a**) Microenvironmental cues (e.g. atRA TGFβ2, BMP7, BMP4) produced by stromal cells that are important in regulating adult stem cell quiescence and tissue differentiation, impose a quiescence phenotype on disseminated solitary tumor cells [1, 8]. This will take place if the DTCs express the proper receptors to sense and respond to the microenvironmental cues [1]. Similarly, specific cues from the microenvironment may lead to reactivation from dormancy [22, 61]. In response to the niche-derived cues DTCs may undergo a set of epigenetic changes that enforce the dormant phenotype. (**b**) Some of these changes (*red*) are also found in senescent cells [92], while others like NR2F1 upregulation [24] are linked to lineage commitment and differentiation during development [76]

Because of the reversible nature of dormancy, it has been proposed that epigenetic changes have a significant role in regulating the onset, maintenance and reactivation from this state [9]. Epigenetics is considered a change in the final biological outcome of a locus or chromosome without changes in the underlying DNA sequence. This is mediated by the post-translational modification of histones (PTMs), ATP-dependent chromatin remodeling, DNA methylation, and the incorporation of specialized histone variants into chromatin. Importantly, cancer is considered a disease consisting of both genetic and epigenetic alterations [10]. Many morphogenetic and microenvironmental cues like retinoic acid, TGFβs and BMPs are known to cause changes in chromatin modification that dictate cell fate and differentiation [11–15]. Importantly, the above-mentioned cues in tissue microenvironments have been also linked to the induction of cancer cell dormancy [16–24] (Fig. 1).

From an evolutionary perspective, there are parallels between dormancy of cancer cells and dormancy phases in organisms [1, 25]. Several lines of evidence from evolutionary and developmental studies suggest that regulation of tumor cell dormancy involves the reciprocal crosstalk between the environment and mechanisms that control transcriptional programs [1, 19, 24, 26–30]. Organisms are known to arrest development in response to stress or nutritional changes [26, 29–32]. For example, in response to oxidative stress or reduced nutrients, *C. elegans* enters a stage called *dauer* during which development is arrested until conditions are propitious [26, 31, 32]. These fate decisions involve specific crosstalk between the microenvironment and transcriptional programs driving the onset and interruption of the *dauer* stage [26]. Similarly in many mammalian species a diapause state is found in blastocysts in response to changes in hormonal levels [33]. An important example can also be found in dormancy of seeds that is controlled by specific signaling and transcriptional programs but only in response to environmental cues [34, 35]. The parallels with DTC dormancy are quite remarkable, suggesting that this phase in cancer is not a rarity but rather a process that recapitulates or taps into evolutionary conserved mechanisms of survival. Given that these are adaptive mechanisms it is clear that inter-conversion between dormant and active states are predominantly plastic in nature.

Despite our progress in understanding cancer cell dormancy, key questions remain open regarding the epigenetic regulation of minimal residual disease (MRD) biology. In this chapter we attempt to address key questions related to this topic using available data or hypothetical scenarios.

- Do dormant residual tumor cells shut down cell cycle progression by modifying their epigenome once they reach a particular microenvironment that stimulates this program?
- Are some tumor cells epigenetically pre-programmed to enable their diaspora to enter dormancy as DTCs?
- Are there specific mutations in chromatin modifiers that affect the rate of dormancy onset and awakening?
- Does every microenvironment remodel the epigenome of residual DTCs in the same way?

Cancer Cell Dormancy within the Dogma of Metastasis

A traditional view of metastasis holds that metastases result from the process of natural selection of tumor cells with metastatic phenotypes [36]. This process is hypothesized to be similar to Darwinian evolution where the genetic changes required for metastasis are stably specified due to genetic mutation. As a result, the metastatic tumor cells are hypothesized to be very rare, not present throughout the bulk of the primary tumor, and to appear late in tumor progression. Darwinian evolution of cancer cell genomes is commonly viewed as a way to generate traits that ultimately propel survival and growth [36]. However, a key feature of Darwinian evolution in the wild is that it selects for adaptation mechanisms that allow for organisms to stop growth to ensure species survival [37–39]. This possibility has not been explored in cancer, but it suggests that dormancy mechanisms might provide a selective advantage to DTC populations.

Through the recent development of new technologies, including sequencing-based mutational and expression profiling, analysis of early dissemination mechanisms, high resolution intravital imaging, and the collection and profiling of disseminated tumor cells (DTC) in animal models and patients [40–43], investigators have challenged the traditional Darwinian model of metastasis. Such studies [44, 45–52] indicate that metastatic ability is acquired at much earlier stages of tumor progression than predicted by the Darwinian model. Importantly, it is clear that DTCs can enter a diapause-like state and remain non-productive or dormant for long periods of time. Intriguingly, this occurs regardless of whether tumor cells carry altered genomes suggesting that microenvironmental and epigenetic mechanisms can dominate over the genetics to drive dormancy [53–55]. The microenvironment and epigenetic model of metastasis opens alternative possibilities to explain clinical phenomena that are not entirely explained by the oncogene-centric view of tumors. For example, why can patients that carry tumors with oncogenic alterations display prolonged disease-free periods with MRD, when these oncogenic alterations should fuel proliferation? The long-lived nature of these phenotypes suggests an epigenetic programming of dormancy fueled by microenvironmental and/or intrinsic cues that have not previously been appreciated [51, 56, 57].

Defining Dormancy States

Three types of dormancy programs have been described in experimental models and these have been reviewed extensively [1, 7, 8] (Table 1). Here we cover the basic definitions for clarity. (1) *Angiogenic dormancy* refers to a stable small tumor mass poorly vascularized that is in a transient equilibrium between cell proliferation and death [1, 25]. Here, an angiogenic switch that leads to enhanced vascularization would promote reactivation of the tumor mass. This dormancy state has not been confirmed in clinical scenarios. (2) *Immune system-induced tumor dormancy* occurs when a tumor mass is kept at a constant size because cytotoxic T-cell-mediated cell death compensates for proliferation in a tumor mass. Evidence of this type of dormancy has been inferred, but not proven, from studies of metastasis arising after organ transplantation [1] and from experimental systems of equilibrium [58, 59]. (3) *Cellular dormancy* defines the state where predominantly single disseminated tumor cells enter a reversible growth arrest that can be induced by several host-derived signals, such as TGFβ2, BMP7, BMP4 or retinoic acid [1, 19, 21, 22, 24].

Table 1 Description of different type of dormancy events

Types of dormancy	Description
Angiogenic dormancy	Small tumor mass poorly vascularized. Proliferation is balanced by cell death caused by insufficient oxygen levels
Immune-mediated dormancy	Small tumor mass or residual cell populations are controlled by cytotoxic T and/or, NK cell mediated cell death that compensates for proliferation. Production of INFγ and TNFα may also induce dormancy (Fig. 1)
Cellular dormancy	Single DTCs enter a reversible growth arrest (quiescence) regulated by lineage commitment transcription factors and G0/G1 arrest machinery. Adult stem cells and senescent cells share gene profiles with dormant cancer cells in experimental models

The three main mechanisms of dormancy defined by experimental systems are indicated. Cellular dormancy is the best characterized mechanistically and validated across multiple labs and has support from the detection of the same genes and proliferation-negative DTCs in clinical samples. The details of mechanisms driving each state have been recently reviewed [1, 8]

While these categories offer some clarity, emerging evidence suggests that some molecules attributed to angiogenic dormancy also function in cellular dormancy, such as thrombospondin [18]. Other scenarios suggests that oncogene inhibition and induction of dormancy is accompanied by an immune regulatory response that sustains the dormancy due to oncogene inactivation [60]. Finally, recent work from the Massague lab showed that Wnt signaling inhibition via DKK1 results in microenvironment-induced quiescence and these cells develop mechanisms to avoid NK cell recognition, thus evading eradication [61]. These data suggest once again that dormancy is initially dominated by microenvironmental signals, such as those that control adult stem cell quiescence [1]. This can happen even if within the same organ there is active expansion of other host cell subpopulations. These programs are followed by immune evasion and vascular niche remodeling [7, 61] changes that support quiescence and survival of DTCs, a main function of dormancy.

There are several clinical scenarios where cellular dormancy is detected. Metastatic dormancy, for instance, happens when DTCs that disseminate from primary tumors have to adapt and survive new microenvironments [1]. In this situation, dormancy at a cellular level is detected in single DTCs isolated from bone marrow of patients with different types of cancer [4, 62, 63]. In addition, metastatic dormancy also occurs during early stages of tumor progression before an overt primary tumor is formed. In this case, several lines of evidence support the notion that early progressed cancer cells that display less evolved genomes, can disseminate and remain as dormant early DTCs at secondary organs [1, 4, 24, 62–64]. This is demonstrated, for example, in DCIS patients where DTCs are found in their bone marrow [42, 43, 62, 65, 66].

Dormancy also occurs as therapy-induced dormancy [67–73] where the treatment used in neoadjuvant or adjuvant settings results in a residual tumor cell population that can persist for long periods of time, depending on the type of tumors and treatments. In these scenarios, dormancy is a mechanism of escape from drug-induced cell death. In this chapter, we will focus primarily on cellular dormancy, as it is best characterized in patients with evidence for epigenetic mechanisms at play.

Microenvironmental Signals Regulate Dormancy

Recent reviews have highlighted the role of microenvironmental signals in controlling DTC behavior [1, 7]. Here we highlight some salient findings that provide a link between the microenvironment and epigenetic mechanisms that we will discuss later in the context of epigenetic mechanisms driving dormancy.

Work from several labs have focused on metastasis-restrictive (e.g. bone marrow, BM) or metastasis-permissive (lung) niches as a way of understanding how the microenvironment might regulate dormancy induction and reactivation [19]. Additional studies showed that DTCs in breast cancer and HNSCC patients and in mouse MMTV-Neu and PyMT models can remain dormant in the BM, but less so in lungs [40, 42, 43, 74]. Using HNSCC and breast cancer models we found that *all-trans* retinoic acid (atRA) and TGFβ2 signaling, which is higher in BM than in lungs, induced a high p38/ERK activity ratio and DTC dormancy [24] (Fig. 1). This work revealed that activation of p38 induced the lineage commitment transcription factor (TF) NR2F1 that orchestrates quiescence/dormancy [24]. NR2F1 is commonly downregulated in cancer tissues, in proliferative primary s.c. (T-HEp3 head and neck squamous cell carcinoma, HNSCC) tumors and lung-derived proliferative DTC lines that readily form metastasis *in vivo* [27, 75]. In contrast, NR2F1 is upregulated in HNSCC cells that are spontaneously dormant s.c. or become dormant in the bone marrow where HNSCC metastasis is exceedingly rare [19]. Moreover, a transcriptomic comparison of dormant BM-HEp3 vs. proliferative T-HEp3 cells [19] revealed that dormant DTCs upregulate atRA regulated genes (RXRα, NR2F1, ALDH1A3, DHRS3, SEMA6B, SEC14L2, ARID5A—unpublished and [24]). Importantly, knock down of NR2F1 in surgery margins, spleen and lung, where cells commonly remain dormant, also awakened dormant residual tumor cells accelerating local recurrences [24]. Surprisingly, NR2F1 knockdown reduced DTCs in the BM suggesting that NR2F1 regulates BM DTC survival. NR2F1 was identified as a lineage commitment regulator and it does so through the regulation of specific enhancers [24, 76]. This work provided the first hints about a microenvironment regulated TF that can remodel chromatin and induce a dormant state. This work will be discussed later with a focus on epigenetic functions.

Others have used powerful gain- and loss-of-function screens to dissect the mechanisms of dormancy regulation. The Giancotti team identified a TGFβ family member, BMP4 as a dormancy inducer, which led to upregulation of p-SMAD levels in DTC nuclei. Expression of the BMP inhibitor Coco/DAND5 reversed BMP signaling and caused reactivation and overt metastasis in lungs [22] (Fig. 1). It was also found that Numb, a Notch inhibitor, also served as an enforcer of dormancy [22, 77]. This suggests that in this model, enhanced BMP signaling and reduced Notch signaling drives dormancy of DTCs in lungs. This highlights how the same microenvironmental signaling themes emerge in models of HNSCC and breast cancer dormancy. As highlighted above, Wnt signaling via DKK1 also results in quiescence of DTCs in models of lung cancer and HER2+ breast cancer. Our work on TGFβ2 revealed that this factor induces long term signaling via SMAD1/5, which are BMP-regulated SMADs [19]. This suggest that BMPs might be induced long term by TGFβ2, and the role of these molecules is reinforced by the findings that both BMP4 and BMP7 induce dormancy [21, 22].

Work focused on understanding how targeted therapies might induce dormancy using unique oncogene-inducible mouse models for Myc, Wnt and ErbB2 revealed that the latter oncogene, when inhibited with drugs or *via* de-induction of a tetracycline-regulated ErbB2 transgene, resulted in the persistence of quiescent residual cells [69, 78]. Early work from the Felsher lab has revealed similar biology when manipulating MYC signaling [70, 71, 79–81]. The ErbB2 work identified Notch1 and c-Met signaling as key in the survival of residual quiescent tumor cells, which was also found in spontaneous dormancy models in HNSCC and TNBC (triple negative breast cancer). In agreement with these studies, it was also found that ErbB1 activation is inhibited in p38^{high} dormant HNSCC cells [82]. These data strongly argue that an imbalance between mitogenic HER1/HER2 signaling *via* ERK1/2 allows for stress signaling *via* p38 to predominate, which can induce dormancy.

An important aspect to discuss is related to understanding how the micro-environmental signals maintain dormancy of DTCs for such prolonged periods. In a recent review, we postulated that just like adult-stem cell quiescence [1], an epigenetic reprogramming sustains the program driven by niche signals. Thus, dormancy of DTCs may follow a pre-established set of rules that evolution has set aside for adult stem cells or other developmental mechanisms when a pause in development or growth would be advantageous (see below). We had also proposed that pathways regulated by organisms like *C. elegans* that pause development in response to certain stress signals would be informative of the mechanisms of dormancy. Importantly, it would be advantageous for cancer cells to follow these rules as it may enable a plasticity capacity that allows for enhanced adaptation. We propose that the microenvironment is key to induce dormancy, but that epigenetic mechanisms stabilize these phenotypes following rules of ontogeny conserved over millions of years of evolution (Fig. 1). From a clinical point of view, one could ask whether induction of a dormant-like epigenome in residual DTCs in permissive microenvironments could overcome the proliferation signals. Further investigation is required to address this possibility.

Epigenetic Regulation of Dormancy Transcriptional Programs

An epigenetic mechanism for the inter-conversion between dormant and malignant states driven by changes in the microenvironment was proposed by Ossowski and Reich more than 30 years ago [83]. In exploring the epigenetic mechanisms that drive dormancy downstream of microenvironmental inputs, our group identified a TF network linked to p38α/β active signaling and dormancy of HNSCC cells [27]. A key epigenetic regulator silenced in dormant cells was DNMT1 accompanied by a large change in a TF network where key G1-S transition TFs were silenced. These included FOXM1, FOXDs, FOXLs, EGR1/2/3, PPARγ, ELK1 and Jun family members among others. These data also revealed that MYC and NFkB activity were silenced in dormant cells although in the case of MYC, the transcript itself was not downregulated [27]. This work also revealed that the TFs p53 and DEC2 were upregulated downstream of p38 signaling, along with NR2F1 and RARβ in dormant tumor cells (Fig. 1). NR2F1 and RARβ are commonly epigenetically silenced in several types of cancer via promoter hyper-methylation. The re-expression of these nuclear receptors in dormancy models suggests that epigenetic regulation can be instrumental in the regulation of these programs. DEC2 is a circadian rhythm regulator with a quiescence induction function in in muscle differentiation that precedes terminal MyoD-driven differentiation [27]. Induction of p53 was consistent with its upstream regulation by p38 and its growth suppressive role [27]. However, the most connected node in the TF network was NR2F1 followed by RARβ and NR1H3. At the time, their function was unclear in dormant cells and the role of NR1H3 remains unknown [27].

Follow up work revealed that atRA [24] upregulated the orphan nuclear receptor and retinoic acid receptor family member NR2F1 as well as RARβ [24]. As mentioned above, NR2F1 was the most highly connected TF node and it shared a large amount of target genes with RARβ [27]. Linking the microenvironment to epigenetic regulation, we showed that NR2F1 regulates chromatin changes associated with a global H3K9me3^{high}/H3K27me3^{high}/H3K4me3^{low} repressive chromatin state [24] (Fig. 1). In local promoter regions, NR2F1 regulated active H3 PTMs on the promoter of its target genes SOX9 and RARβ [24]. Recent analysis of H3 PTMs that mark active and poised enhancers (H3K4me1/H3K27ac active, H3K4me1 only, poised), is improving our understanding of NR2F1-regulated programs and revealed that many genes induced in dormant cells are regulated by active enhancers containing binding elements regulated by NR2F1 and other key TFs controlling G0/G1 exit (unpublished and [76]).

Dormancy could be induced by a combination treatment with 5-azacytidine and atRA, suggesting that the global chromatin repressive state can be activated in malignant cells. Similar results on reprogramming of dormancy were published by others using different strategies. For example, treatment with 5-azacytidine as a single agent resulted in decreased expression of G0/G1 exit genes including DNMT1 and FOXM1 in hematological and epithelial tumor cells [84]. Interestingly, other genes that are induced by p38 signaling in dormant HNSCC cells [27, 85], such as RARβ and CDKN1A were induced by 5-azacytidine [84]. Epigenetic modulation of DTC fate may be achieved with other drugs that affect chromatin modifying enzymes, such as histone deacetylases (HDACs). In uveal melanoma models, HDAC inhibitors, such as LBH-589, reprogrammed uveal melanoma lines from a high metastatic risk (Class 2) to a low risk (Class 1) state [86]. This reprogramming was accompanied by induction of G0/G1 arrest and the activation of gene programs that resembled melanocytic differentiation. We propose that HDAC inhibitors and/or DNA demethylating agents might represent alternative therapies to induce dormancy of uveal melanoma or other cancer cell types. It is also possible that demethylating agents or HDAC inhibitors coupled to specific RARα, NR2F1, RARβ agonists or with specific inhibitors of FOXM1 or DNMT1 could be used to reprogram tumor cells into dormancy. As we identify the key chromatin factors important to target for dormancy induction, we may identify drugs that specifically target chromatin factors that, in combination with other targeted therapies, may allow reprograming cells into dormancy and prevent relapse.

Repressive chromatin has been linked to the histone variant macroH2A, which is involved in gene silencing in senescent, differentiating and quiescent cells [87–90] and also found upregulated at the mRNA level in dormant HEp3 cells in response to p38 activation [27]. Proliferation of melanoma cells has also been linked to upregulation of H2A.Z.2 histone variant [91]. Interestingly this histone variant is downregulated in dormant HNSCC cells [27], suggesting that differential regulation of histone variants is key to establish the dormant phenotype (Fig. 1).

It has also been shown that proteolytic cleavage of histone H3.3, which occurs during senescence [92] is also found in quiescent cells [92–94]. The cleaved form of H3.3 is associated with inactive promoters of cell cycle genes in senescent cells [92]. Thus, dormant cells may tap into similar programs of growth arrest as quiescent and senescent cells that allows for a long-lived growth arrest. Whether such proteolytic processing of histone H3.3 can be stimulated by microenvironmental cues and whether this is true in dormant DTCs in patients is unknown. Surprisingly, senescent fibroblasts induced by oncogenic stress or by overexpression of a cleaved form of histone H3.3 were found to upregulate TGFβ2 and BMP4, two micro-environmental cues found to induce dormancy [19, 22, 92]. These data argue that deep growth arrest accompanied by a strong epigenetic remodeling of the chromatin and alteration of gene expression, are likely to require the sustained signaling from microenvironmental cues to maintain the phenotype (Fig. 1).

Further linking epigenetic regulation to dormancy regulation, a recent loss of function screen to identify dormancy 'enforcers' revealed that the histone methyl-transferase Smyd5, which trimethylates H4K20 (repressive mark) is required for lung DTC dormancy [77] (Fig. 1). Furthermore, the long non-coding RNA MALAT1 (metastasis-associated lung adenocarcinoma transcript 1) is a mediator of meta-static reactivation in the lung [77]. These data together suggest that specific TFs, histone variants, chromatin modifiers and non-coding RNAs are important regula-tors of epigenetic programs linked to dormancy. Molecularly defining the epigenetic dormancy mechanisms and how they play into late cancer relapse is an essential outstanding question in cancer dormancy research.

Transcriptional Programs in Adult Stem Cells and Dormant Cancer Cells

Recent publications suggest that dormancy of DTCs may be regulated by some of the same rules that regulate adult stem cell biology [1, 19, 21, 22, 24]. Remarkably, there are several similarities between adult stem cells, embryonic stem cells and dormant residual tumor cells. In adult stem cells, for instance, around 60% of induced genes overlap with genes upregulated and previously described during the dormancy state of tumor cells [1, 95]. In addition, post-surgery residual dormant cells were found to induce the pluripotency core NANOG, SOX2 and OCT4 [24]. In this scenario, at least NANOG was required to maintain quiescence of BM DTCs [24]. Remarkably, these master TFs regulate enhancers and epigenetic modifications (Boyer 2005) during embryonic development suggesting that similar functions may occur during dormancy state. Is it possible that dormant cells express these ESC TFs to maintain their epig-enome in a plastic state that would allow for reactivation despite activating deep quies-cence programs?

Another feature found in dormant DTCs is the downregulation of a network of genes regulated by c-Myc [24, 27]. This was also recently reported in ESCs where Myc depletion induced a reversible pluripotent diapause-like state [33]. This state was char-acterized by a deep growth arrest, but maintenance of the expression of pluripotency TFs Nanog, Sox2 and Oct4 [33]. A similar link was previously observed in BM-derived dormant cells or cells that reprogram into dormancy in response to reduced ERK1/2 and active p38 signaling [24, 96]. These findings indicate that by downregulating Myc activity, dormant tumor cells and naïve ESC enter a reversible cell cycle arrest. However, they maintain an undifferentiated state and reactivation capacity, albeit with different fates, which is mediated by the pluripotency core TFs. This differential regula-tion of pluripotency and proliferation programs was highlighted by Orkin et al. [97], and suggests that the reversible nature of cells in diapause or dormancy may rely on the plasticity of epigenetic programs enabled by the pluripotency TFs. Along these lines, retinal Muller stem cells require SOX2 to maintain quiescence through the Notch1 pathway as well as self-renewal capacity [98]. The Notch1 pathway was also linked to dormancy induced after targeting the HER2 oncogene [67] and JAG1 and HES1 upregulation were linked to NR2F1 regulated dormancy in HNSCC cells [24], arguing for a function of Notch signaling during residual cancer cell dormancy. These studies suggested that juxtacrine signaling between tumor cells or with host cells may regulate these epigenetic programs that result in quiescence and/or survival of DTCs.

Transcriptional Programs in Dormant Residual Disease in Patients

The concept of dormancy or mitotic arrest was first described by Willis and then Hadfield in the 1940s and 50s [4, 99]. In the clinic, it refers to the period of time after primary tumor treatment where single tumor cells or small clusters of tumor cells remain undetectable and quiescent for several years and patients present no symptoms of disease [25].

DTCs may reside in multiple organs and evidence of metastatic disease after organ transplantation has served as evidence that residual disease can go undetected for long periods [1]. These transplantation studies also revealed that changes in the immune microenvironment can lead to reactivation of DTCs [1]. However, this clinical situation does not allow the capture of disease during the dormancy phase. Thus, investigators have resorted to detection of DTCs in the bone marrow and lymph nodes or to detect circulating tumor cells (CTCs). Detection of DTCs in BM aspirates from post-surgery asymptomatic and symptomatic patients can predict relapses in different organs [100]. Even the detection of as little as 1 DTC in the BM predicts poor prognosis [100]. However, relapse can occur a few years or many years after surgery. This argues that isolating and detecting the gene expression profile of these cells may allow the determination of whether they are in a dormant or reactivated state.

Genetic and transcriptomic profiling of DTCs in metastasis negative or M0 patients may prove useful to identify targets for which drugs are available and also to discover new mechanisms. This is illustrated by the discovery that HER2 is more frequently amplified in DTCs from esophageal cancer patients, an alteration rarely observed in the primary lesions [40]. Transcriptomic analyses may also provide evidence of transcriptional programs associated with dormancy. Accordingly, the group of Morrisey was the first to show the dormancy status of BM DTCs and the correlation with clinical dormancy. In this work, 42.8–47% of residual DTCs from prostate cancer patients with no evidence of disease (NED) after surgery showed NR2F1, TGFβ2 and BMP7 upregulation vs. 10.3% in advance metastatic disease (ADV) patient-derived DTCs [5]. In addition, the genes induced in the dormancy signature identified downstream of p38 signaling, were also enriched in these DTCs from NED patients [64]. Enrichment for the p38 signaling pathway in the genes expressed in dormant NED patient-derived DTCs was also confirmed independently of the p38-regulated dormancy signature [85] and this identified additional p38 target genes linked to dormancy in patients [64].

These results reveal not only that the mechanisms of dormancy can be mapped to human DTCs, but also that genes such as NR2F1 or others in the dormancy signature, may serve as markers to identify dormant DTCs.

Conclusions

Understanding dormancy of cancer cells opens an incredible opportunity to prevent metastasis by enforcing the quiescence programs or by inducing cell death in residual tumor cells. Exploration of the epigenetic mechanisms driving dormancy is key to achieve such goals. Chromatin modifiers can be targeted pharmacologically offering an opportunity to enhance or block programs that induce dormancy or dormant cancer cell survival, respectively. It will be important to functionalize the role of the epigenetic regulators found in the various models and validate their expression and function in human DTCs. As mentioned above, the complementary approach of directly interrogating the epigenome of residual DTCs in patients from distinct organ sites will provide an unbiased and exceptional opportunity to understand how the epigenome is reprogrammed during the different stages of cancer progression. Advances in single cell genomics and epigenome analysis will surely allow researchers to probe these important questions in the near future.

References

1. Sosa MS, Bragado P, Aguirre-Ghiso JA (2014) Mechanisms of disseminated cancer cell dormancy: an awakening field. Nat Rev Cancer 14:611–622. doi:10.1038/nrc3793
2. Aguirre-Ghiso JA, Bragado P, Sosa MS (2013) Metastasis awakening: targeting dormant cancer. Nat Med 19:276–277. doi:10.1038/nm.3120
3. Polzer B, Klein CA (2013) Metastasis awakening: the challenges of targeting minimal residual cancer. Nat Med 19:274–275. doi:10.1038/nm.3121
4. Klein CA (2010) Framework models of tumor dormancy from patient-derived observations. Curr Opin Genet Dev 21:42–49
5. Chéry L et al (2014) Characterization of single disseminated prostate cancer cells reveals tumor cell heterogeneity and identifies dormancy associated pathways. Oncotarget 5(20):9939–9951
6. Ossowski L, Aguirre-Ghiso JA (2010) Dormancy of metastatic melanoma. Pigment Cell Melanoma Res 23:41–56. doi:10.1111/j.1755-148X.2009.00647.x
7. Ghajar CM (2015) Metastasis prevention by targeting the dormant niche. Nat Rev Cancer 15:238–247. doi:10.1038/nrc3910
8. Giancotti FG (2013) Mechanisms governing metastatic dormancy and reactivation. Cell 155:750–764. doi:10.1016/j.cell.2013.10.029
9. Crea F, Nur Saidy NR, Collins CC, Wang Y (2015) The epigenetic/noncoding origin of tumor dormancy. Trends Mol Med 21:206–211. doi:10.1016/j.molmed.2015.02.005
10. Vardabasso C et al (2014) Histone variants: emerging players in cancer biology. Cell Mol Life Sci 71:379–404. doi:10.1007/s00018-013-1343-z
11. Wilkinson DS et al (2005) A direct intersection between p53 and transforming growth factor beta pathways targets chromatin modification and transcription repression of the alpha-fetoprotein gene. Mol Cell Biol 25:1200–1212. doi:10.1128/MCB.25.3.1200-1212.2005

12. Glenisson W, Castronovo V, Waltregny D (2007) Histone deacetylase 4 is required for TGFbeta1-induced myofibroblastic differentiation. Biochim Biophys Acta 1773:1572–1582. doi:10.1016/j.bbamcr.2007.05.016
13. Jepsen K et al (2007) SMRT-mediated repression of an H3K27 demethylase in progression from neural stem cell to neuron. Nature 450:415–419. doi:10.1038/nature06270
14. Cras A et al (2007) Epigenetic patterns of the retinoic acid receptor beta2 promoter in retinoic acid-resistant thyroid cancer cells. Oncogene 26:4018–4024. doi:10.1038/sj.onc.1210178
15. Yang D, Okamura H, Nakashima Y, Haneji T (2013) Histone demethylase Jmjd3 regulates osteoblast differentiation via transcription factors Runx2 and osterix. J Biol Chem 288:33530–33541. doi:10.1074/jbc.M113.497040
16. Yumoto K, Eber MR, Berry JE, Taichman RS, Shiozawa Y (2014) Molecular pathways: niches in metastatic dormancy. Clin Cancer Res. doi:10.1158/1078-0432.CCR-13-0897
17. Ruppender NS, Morrissey C, Lange PH, Vessella RL (2013) Dormancy in solid tumors: implications for prostate cancer. Cancer Metastasis Rev 32:501–509. doi:10.1007/s10555-013-9422-z
18. Ghajar CM et al (2013) The perivascular niche regulates breast tumour dormancy. Nat Cell Biol 15:807–817. doi:10.1038/ncb2767
19. Bragado P et al (2013) TGF-beta2 dictates disseminated tumour cell fate in target organs through TGF-beta-RIII and p38alpha/beta signalling. Nat Cell Biol 15:1351–1361. doi:10.1038/ncb2861
20. Boyerinas B et al (2013) Adhesion to osteopontin in the bone marrow niche regulates lymphoblastic leukemia cell dormancy. Blood 121:4821–4831. doi:10.1182/blood-2012-12-475483
21. Kobayashi A et al (2011) Bone morphogenetic protein 7 in dormancy and metastasis of prostate cancer stem-like cells in bone. J Exp Med 208:2641–2655. doi:10.1084/jem.20110840
22. Gao H et al (2012) The BMP inhibitor coco reactivates breast cancer cells at lung metastatic sites. Cell 150:764–779. doi:10.1016/j.cell.2012.06.035
23. Sosa MS (2016) Dormancy programs as emerging antimetastasis therapeutic alternatives. Mol Cell Oncol 3:e1029062. doi:10.1080/23723556.2015.1029062
24. Sosa MS et al (2015) NR2F1 controls tumour cell dormancy via SOX9- and RARbeta-driven quiescence programmes. Nat Commun 6:6170. doi:10.1038/ncomms7170
25. Aguirre-Ghiso JA (2007) Models, mechanisms and clinical evidence for cancer dormancy. Nat Rev Cancer 7:834–846. doi:10.1038/nrc2256
26. Wang J, Kim SK (2003) Global analysis of dauer gene expression in Caenorhabditis elegans. Development 130:1621–1634
27. Adam AP et al (2009) Computational identification of a p38SAPK-regulated transcription factor network required for tumor cell quiescence. Cancer Res 69:5664–5672. doi:10.1158/0008-5472.CAN-08-3820
28. Yamazaki S et al (2009) TGF-beta as a candidate bone marrow niche signal to induce hematopoietic stem cell hibernation. Blood 113:1250–1256
29. Frerichs KU et al (1998) Suppression of protein synthesis in brain during hibernation involves inhibition of protein initiation and elongation. Proc Natl Acad Sci U S A 95:14511–14516
30. Frerichs KU, Hallenbeck JM (1998) Hibernation in ground squirrels induces state and species-specific tolerance to hypoxia and aglycemia: an in vitro study in hippocampal slices. J Cereb Blood Flow Metab 18:168–175
31. Fukuyama M, Rougvie AE, Rothman JH (2006) C. elegans DAF-18/PTEN mediates nutrient-dependent arrest of cell cycle and growth in the germline. Curr Biol 16:773–779
32. Melendez A et al (2003) Autophagy genes are essential for dauer development and life-span extension in C. elegans. Science 301:1387–1391
33. Scognamiglio R et al (2016) Myc depletion induces a pluripotent dormant state mimicking diapause. Cell 164:668–680. doi:10.1016/j.cell.2015.12.033
34. Gao F, Ayele BT (2014) Functional genomics of seed dormancy in wheat: advances and prospects. Front Plant Sci 5:458. doi:10.3389/fpls.2014.00458

35. Chinnusamy V, Gong Z, Zhu JK (2008) Abscisic acid-mediated epigenetic processes in plant development and stress responses. J Integr Plant Biol 50:1187–1195. doi:10.1111/j.1744-7909.2008.00727.x
36. Hanahan D, Weinberg RA (2011) Hallmarks of cancer: the next generation. Cell 144:646–674. doi:10.1016/j.cell.2011.02.013
37. Scott MF, Otto SP (2014) Why wait? Three mechanisms selecting for environment-dependent developmental delays. J Evol Biol 27:2219–2232. doi:10.1111/jeb.12474
38. Seifan M, Seifan T, Schiffers K, Jeltsch F, Tielborger K (2013) Beyond the competition-colonization trade-off: linking multiple trait response to disturbance characteristics. Am Nat 181:151–160. doi:10.1086/668844
39. Flatt T, Amdam GV, Kirkwood TB, Omholt SW (2013) Life-history evolution and the polyphenic regulation of somatic maintenance and survival. Q Rev Biol 88:185–218
40. Stoecklein NH et al (2008) Direct genetic analysis of single disseminated cancer cells for prediction of outcome and therapy selection in esophageal cancer. Cancer Cell 13:441–453. doi:10.1016/j.ccr.2008.04.005
41. Klein CA (2008) The direct molecular analysis of metastatic precursor cells in breast cancer: a chance for a better understanding of metastasis and for personalised medicine. Eur J Cancer 44:2721–2725
42. Husemann Y et al (2008) Systemic spread is an early step in breast cancer. Cancer Cell 13:58–68. doi:10.1016/j.ccr.2007.12.003
43. Schardt JA et al (2005) Genomic analysis of single cytokeratin-positive cells from bone marrow reveals early mutational events in breast cancer. Cancer Cell 8:227–239. doi:10.1016/j.ccr.2005.08.003
44. Mantovani A, Giavazzi R, Alessandri G, Spreafico F, Garattini S (1981) Characterization of tumor lines derived from spontaneous metastases of a transplanted murine sarcoma. Eur J Cancer 17:71–76
45. Giavazzi R, Alessandri G, Spreafico F, Garattini S, Mantovani A (1980) Metastasizing capacity of tumour cells from spontaneous metastases of transplanted murine tumours. Br J Cancer 42:462–472
46. Milas L, Peters LJ, Ito H (1983) Spontaneous metastasis: random or selective? Clin Exp Metastasis 1:309–315
47. Wyckoff J et al (2004) A paracrine loop between tumor cells and macrophages is required for tumor cell migration in mammary tumors. Cancer Res 64:7022–7029
48. van't Veer LJ et al (2002) Gene expression profiling predicts clinical outcome of breast cancer. Nature 415:530–536
49. Ramaswamy S, Ross KN, Lander ES, Golub TR (2003) A molecular signature of metastasis in primary solid tumors. Nat Genet 33:49–54. doi:10.1038/ng1060
50. Wang W et al (2004) Identification and testing of a gene expression signature of invasive carcinoma cells within primary mammary tumors. Cancer Res 64:8585–8594. doi:10.1158/0008-5472.CAN-04-1136
51. Wang W et al (2005) Tumor cells caught in the act of invading: their strategy for enhanced cell motility. Trends Cell Biol 15:138–145. doi:10.1016/j.tcb.2005.01.003
52. Wang W et al (2007) Coordinated regulation of pathways for enhanced cell motility and chemotaxis is conserved in rat and mouse mammary tumors. Cancer Res 67:3505–3511. doi:10.1158/0008-5472.CAN-06-3714
53. Kitzis A et al (2001) Persistence of transcriptionally silent BCR-ABL rearrangements in chronic myeloid leukemia patients in sustained complete cytogenetic remission. Leuk Lymphoma 42:933–944. doi:10.3109/10428190109097712
54. Chomel JC et al (2000) Persistence of BCR-ABL genomic rearrangement in chronic myeloid leukemia patients in complete and sustained cytogenetic remission after interferon-alpha therapy or allogeneic bone marrow transplantation. Blood 95:404–408
55. Talpaz M et al (1994) Persistence of dormant leukemic progenitors during interferon-induced remission in chronic myelogenous leukemia. Analysis by polymerase chain reaction of individual colonies. J Clin Invest 94:1383–1389. doi:10.1172/JCI117473

56. Condeelis J, Singer RH, Segall JE (2005) The great escape: when cancer cells hijack the genes for chemotaxis and motility. Annu Rev Cell Dev Biol 21:695–718. doi:10.1146/annurev.cellbio.21.122303.120306
57. Bissell MJ, Radisky D (2001) Putting tumours in context. Nat Rev Cancer 1:46–54. doi:10.1038/35094059
58. Koebel CM et al (2007) Adaptive immunity maintains occult cancer in an equilibrium state. Nature 450:903–907
59. Matzavinos A, Chaplain MA, Kuznetsov VA (2004) Mathematical modelling of the spatio-temporal response of cytotoxic T-lymphocytes to a solid tumour. Math Med Biol 21:1–34
60. Rakhra K et al (2010) CD4(+) T cells contribute to the remodeling of the microenvironment required for sustained tumor regression upon oncogene inactivation. Cancer Cell 18:485–498. doi:10.1016/j.ccr.2010.10.002
61. Malladi S et al (2016) Metastatic latency and immune evasion through autocrine inhibition of WNT. Cell 165:45–60. doi:10.1016/j.cell.2016.02.025
62. Guzvic M, Klein CA (2013) Cancer dormancy: time to explore its clinical relevance. Breast Cancer Res 15:321. doi:10.1186/bcr3590
63. Klein CA (2008) The direct molecular analysis of metastatic precursor cells in breast cancer: a chance for a better understanding of metastasis and for personalised medicine. Eur J Cancer 44:2721–2725. doi:10.1016/j.ejca.2008.09.035
64. Chery L et al (2014) Characterization of single disseminated prostate cancer cells reveals tumor cell heterogeneity and identifies dormancy associated pathways. Oncotarget 5:9939–9951. doi:10.18632/oncotarget.2480
65. Fehm T et al (2008) Tumor cell dormancy: implications for the biology and treatment of breast cancer. APMIS 116:742–753. doi:10.1111/j.1600-0463.2008.01047.x
66. Klein CA, Holzel D (2006) Systemic cancer progression and tumor dormancy: mathematical models meet single cell genomics. Cell Cycle 5:1788–1798
67. Abravanel DL et al (2015) Notch promotes recurrence of dormant tumor cells following HER2/neu-targeted therapy. J Clin Invest 125:2484–2496. doi:10.1172/JCI74883
68. Moody SE et al (2005) The transcriptional repressor snail promotes mammary tumor recurrence. Cancer Cell 8:197–209
69. Moody SE et al (2002) Conditional activation of Neu in the mammary epithelium of transgenic mice results in reversible pulmonary metastasis. Cancer Cell 2:451–461
70. Giuriato S et al (2006) Sustained regression of tumors upon MYC inactivation requires p53 or thrombospondin-1 to reverse the angiogenic switch. Proc Natl Acad Sci U S A 103:16266–16271. doi:10.1073/pnas.0608017103
71. Shachaf CM et al (2004) MYC inactivation uncovers pluripotent differentiation and tumour dormancy in hepatocellular cancer. Nature 431:1112–1117
72. Adomako A et al (2015) Identification of markers that functionally define a quiescent multiple myeloma cell sub-population surviving bortezomib treatment. BMC Cancer 15:444. doi:10.1186/s12885-015-1460-1
73. Schewe DM, Aguirre-Ghiso JA (2009) Inhibition of eIF2alpha dephosphorylation maximizes bortezomib efficiency and eliminates quiescent multiple myeloma cells surviving proteasome inhibitor therapy. Cancer Res 69:1545–1552. doi:10.1158/0008-5472.CAN-08-3858
74. Stoecklein NH, Klein CA (2010) Genetic disparity between primary tumours, disseminated tumour cells, and manifest metastasis. Int J Cancer 126:589–598. doi:10.1002/ijc.24916
75. Aguirre-Ghiso JA, Ossowski L, Rosenbaum SK (2004) Green fluorescent protein tagging of extracellular signal-regulated kinase and p38 pathways reveals novel dynamics of pathway activation during primary and metastatic growth. Cancer Res 64:7336–7345. doi:10.1158/0008-5472.CAN-04-0113
76. Rada-Iglesias A et al (2012) Epigenomic annotation of enhancers predicts transcriptional regulators of human neural crest. Cell Stem Cell 11:633–648
77. Gao H et al (2014) Forward genetic screens in mice uncover mediators and suppressors of metastatic reactivation. Proc Natl Acad Sci U S A 111:16532–16537. doi:10.1073/pnas.1403234111

78. Alvarez JV et al (2013) Par-4 downregulation promotes breast cancer recurrence by preventing multinucleation following targeted therapy. Cancer Cell 24:30–44. doi:10.1016/j.ccr.2013.05.007
79. Felsher DW (2008) Oncogene addiction versus oncogene amnesia: perhaps more than just a bad habit? Cancer Res 68:3081–3086. doi:10.1158/0008-5472.CAN-07-5832. discussion 3086, 68/9/3081 [pii]
80. Jain M et al (2002) Sustained loss of a neoplastic phenotype by brief inactivation of MYC. Science 297:102–104
81. Felsher DW, Bishop JM (1999) Reversible tumorigenesis by MYC in hematopoietic lineages. Mol Cell 4:199–207
82. Liu D, Aguirre Ghiso J, Estrada Y, Ossowski L (2002) EGFR is a transducer of the urokinase receptor initiated signal that is required for in vivo growth of a human carcinoma. Cancer Cell 1:445–457
83. Ossowski L, Reich E (1983) Changes in malignant phenotype of a human carcinoma conditioned by growth environment. Cell 33:323–333
84. Tsai HC et al (2012) Transient low doses of DNA-demethylating agents exert durable antitumor effects on hematological and epithelial tumor cells. Cancer Cell 21:430–446
85. Kim RS et al (2012) Dormancy signatures and metastasis in estrogen receptor positive and negative breast cancer. PLoS One 7:e35569. doi:10.1371/journal.pone.0035569
86. Landreville S et al (2012) Histone deacetylase inhibitors induce growth arrest and differentiation in uveal melanoma. Clin Cancer Res 18:408–416. doi:10.1158/1078-0432.CCR-11-0946
87. Kapoor A et al (2010) The histone variant macroH2A suppresses melanoma progression through regulation of CDK8. Nature 468:1105–1109. doi:10.1038/nature09590
88. Bernstein E et al (2008) A phosphorylated subpopulation of the histone variant macroH2A1 is excluded from the inactive X chromosome and enriched during mitosis. Proc Natl Acad Sci U S A 105:1533–1538. doi:10.1073/pnas.0711632105
89. Zhang R et al (2005) Formation of MacroH2A-containing senescence-associated heterochromatin foci and senescence driven by ASF1a and HIRA. Dev Cell 8:19–30. doi:10.1016/j.devcel.2004.10.019. S1534580704004083 [pii]
90. Gaspar-Maia A et al (2013) MacroH2A histone variants act as a barrier upon reprogramming towards pluripotency. Nat Commun 4:1565
91. Vardabasso C et al (2015) Histone variant H2A.Z.2 mediates proliferation and drug sensitivity of malignant melanoma. Mol Cell 59:75–88. doi:10.1016/j.molcel.2015.05.009
92. Duarte LF et al (2014) Histone H3.3 and its proteolytically processed form drive a cellular senescence programme. Nat Commun 5:5210. doi:10.1038/ncomms6210
93. Duncan EM et al (2008) Cathepsin L proteolytically processes histone H3 during mouse embryonic stem cell differentiation. Cell 135:284–294. doi:10.1016/j.cell.2008.09.055
94. Allis CD, Bowen JK, Abraham GN, Glover CV, Gorovsky MA (1980) Proteolytic processing of histone H3 in chromatin: a physiologically regulated event in Tetrahymena micronuclei. Cell 20:55–64
95. Cheung TH, Rando TA (2013) Molecular regulation of stem cell quiescence. Nat Rev Mol Cell Biol 14:329–340. doi:10.1038/nrm3591
96. Aguirre-Ghiso JA, Liu D, Mignatti A, Kovalski K, Ossowski L (2001) Urokinase receptor and fibronectin regulate the ERK(MAPK) to p38(MAPK) activity ratios that determine carcinoma cell proliferation or dormancy in vivo. Mol Biol Cell 12:863–879
97. Kim J, Chu J, Shen X, Wang J, Orkin SH (2008) An extended transcriptional network for pluripotency of embryonic stem cells. Cell 132:1049–1061. doi:10.1016/j.cell.2008.02.039
98. Taranova OV et al (2006) SOX2 is a dose-dependent regulator of retinal neural progenitor competence. Genes Dev 20:1187–1202. doi:10.1101/gad.1407906
99. Hadfield G (1954) The dormant cancer cell. Br Med J 2:607–610
100. Braun S et al (2005) A pooled analysis of bone marrow micrometastasis in breast cancer. N Engl J Med 353:793–802

Biological and Clinical Evidence for Metabolic Dormancy in Solid Tumors Post Therapy

Noushin Nabavi, Susan L. Ettinger, Francesco Crea,
Yuzhuo Wang, and Colin C. Collins

Abstract Despite many advances in the understanding of cancer biology, patient survival has only modestly improved over the past few decades. This is partly due to the dismissal of an important phase of cancer progression called therapy-induced dormancy which arises during the course of (neo)adjuvant therapy. This review describes recent efforts in understanding the mechanisms that 'dormant' cancer cells adopt to survive and develop resistance prior to their relapse into secondary tumors. The focus is particularly on metabolic reprogramming that ensues as a consequence of tumor adaptation to therapy.

Keywords Metabolic dormancy • Solid tumors • Tumor *dormancy* • Metabolism • Therapy induced tumor resistance • Therapy induced dormancy

Noushin Nabavi and Susan L. Ettinger are co-first authors.

N. Nabavi • Y. Wang (✉)
Department of Experimental Therapeutics and Department of Urologic Sciences,
BC Cancer Agency and University of British Columbia, Vancouver, BC, Canada
e-mail: nnabavi@prostatecentre.com; ywang@bccrc.ca

S.L. Ettinger
Laboratory for Advanced Genome Analysis, Vancouver Prostate Centre,
Vancouver, BC, Canada

Department of Urologic Sciences, University of British Columbia, Vancouver, BC, Canada

F. Crea
School of Life, Health & Chemical Sciences, The Open University, Walton Hall, Milton
Keynes, Buckinghamshire, UK

C.C. Collins (✉)
Laboratory for Advanced Genome Analysis, Vancouver Prostate Centre, 2660 Oak St,
Vancouver, BC, Canada, V6H 3Z6

Department of Urologic Sciences, University of British Columbia, 2329 West Mall,
Vancouver, BC, Canada, V6T 1Z4
e-mail: ccollins@prostatecentre.com

© Springer International Publishing AG 2017
Y. Wang, F. Crea (eds.), *Tumor Dormancy and Recurrence*, Cancer Drug
Discovery and Development, DOI 10.1007/978-3-319-59242-8_2

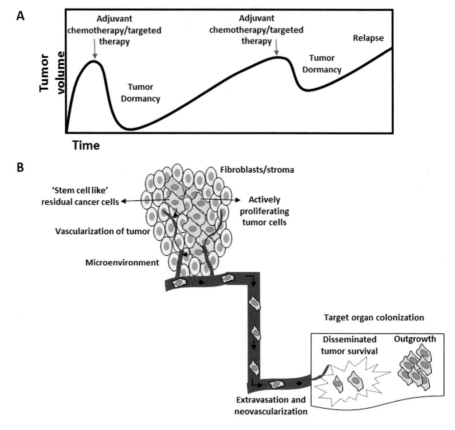

Fig. 1 (**a**) The clinical course of a majority of cancer types initiating with an increasing tumor burden until treatment with first (neo)adjuvant chemotherapy or targeted therapy. The dormancy phase ensues upon reduction of tumors to a minimum size before emergence as therapy resistant tumor. (**b**) Cancer cell's metastatic dissemination in distant organs through extravasation and neo-vascularization of new tissues

Introduction

Tumor dormancy is signified by the period in cancer progression during which there is a minimal residual disease-state as a consequence of surgical resection or neo-adjuvant treatment of primary tumors and prior to relapse either locally or in distant organs (Fig. 1a). Tumor dormancy post-therapy ensues when proliferation is counter-balanced by apoptosis, and the transition has been ascribed to four main attributes: (i) angiogenic dormancy, (ii) immunologic dormancy, (iii) micrometa-static dormancy, and (iv) dormancy regulation through microenvironmental factors [1]. Cellular dormancy occurs when cancer cells transition to a stem-cell like revers-ible growth arrest phase following treatment, the mechanisms of which are poorly understood. These quiescent residual dormant cells must acquire profound genetic or epigenetic reprogramming that allow them to escape immunosurveillance, and help them adapt to an unwelcoming microenvironment in order to relapse. Whether these are cancer stem cells is still an active topic of debate in many cancer fields.

Hence, dormancy is an important phase to consider clinically because patient mortality is often due to the permanence of residual tumor cells (RTCs) or disseminated tumor cells (DTCs) that are highly resistant to therapy and capable of generating metastatic and incurable diseases. Circulating tumor cells (CTCs), on the other hand, are associated with active and metastatic malignancies [2] and distinct from the former two (Fig. 1b). The 'seed and soil' hypothesis of 'tumor and stroma' interactions account for relapse and metastasis of tumors that eventually cause a majority of patient deaths in many cancer types [3]. This is important because the expression of many of the tumor suppressors and oncogenes is context-dependent and require specific tissue microenvironments to exert their functions [4].

Considering the conflicting clinical results and logistical challenges in addressing tumor dormancy, animal models that closely recapitulate the clinical discourse of cancer are incredibly valuable [5–9]. Use of post-treatment patient-derived xenograft models allow one to rule out the confounding metabolic adaptations typically found *in vitro* models due to tissue culture conditions.

Some of the challenging questions that remain to be investigated include the causes of dormant cancer cell re-awakening, distinctions and similarities of various dormant cancer types, and the dormant cancer cell signature of long-term versus short-term patient survivors.

Here, we introduce 'metabolic dormancy' in the context of cancer. Previously, this term has been used to describe aquatic invertebrates (e.g. Caenorhabditis elegans) entering a state of developmental and metabolic dormancy for coping with their extreme environmental conditions [10]. In microbiology, metabolic dormancy has been used to describe Mycobacterium avium's evolved response to starvation [11]. *E. coli* and *S. cerevisiae* also enter a stationary phase during which the metabolism of carbohydrates, amino acids, and phospholipids are considerably reduced [12] under the close regulation of reactive oxygen species (ROS) and superoxide dismutases, MTOR, and stress response transcription factors [13, 14]. Metabolic dormancy in the context of cancer is attributed to a reprogramming and switch in metabolism during dormancy in order to use a minimum supply of energy for survival either at the site of origin, as minimal residual disease post-treatment, or in a new microenvironmental niche occupied by disseminated dormant tumor cells. Since the bone marrow acts as the recipient organ of many cancer cell metastases (dissemination to the bone), understanding the hematopoietic stem cells niche of the bone marrow is also essential [15–17]. Therefore, it is not surprising that many different mechanisms need to converge in order to result in maintenance of quiescence (Fig. 2).

Thus, there exists an urgent need for identifying the effective survival strategies of dormant cancer cells and for determining prognostic and diagnostic markers of specific cancers. The ultimate aim of this chapter is to evaluate recent findings that intervene in progression, and metastatic relapse of cancer, targeting the energetics switch of cancer cells after therapy. Understanding the intricate biology of dormant tumors and metabolic mechanisms that lead to their switch from dormancy to relapse into secondary tumors are critical steps towards designing therapeutic strategies.

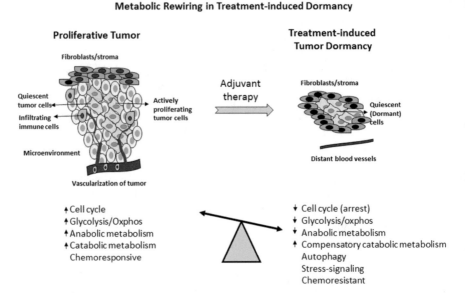

Fig. 2 Comparison between properties of proliferative active tumors and quiescent treatment induced dormant tumors. A heterogeneous mass of proliferative tumors exhibit increased cell cycle, anabolic and catabolic metabolism to supply energy for growth. Other attributes include chemoresponsiveness and vascularization. Dormant tumors, on the other hand, exhibit lowered cycling and metabolic activities to support their survival. Other attributes include development of chemoresistance and profound genetic/epigenetic reprogramming

The Derangement of Metabolic Wiring in Cancer

In the presence of oxygen, most normal tissues derive their energy by metabolizing glucose to pyruvate through glycolysis, and then oxidize the majority of the generated pyruvate to carbon dioxide in the mitochondria through the tricarboxylic acid (TCA) cycle coupled to oxidative phosphorylation (OXPHOS) [18]. Under anaerobic conditions, normal cells redirect the pyruvate generated from glycolysis away from oxphos towards lactate production [19]. The fundamental paradigm shift that Otto Warburg proposed was that in contrast to normal cells, rapidly proliferating cancer cells rewire their metabolic programming and switch to accelerated aerobic glycolysis and lactate production [20]. Recent studies now show that in addition to high rates of glucose metabolism, some cancer cells can maintain high rates of oxphos as well [21]. The process of aerobic glycolysis is more rapid than oxphos and while it provides the increased rate of ATP production required for increased cell division it also diverts glucose into anabolic biosynthetic pathways upstream of pyruvate production [22] required for the vital replication of cellular biomass. These anabolic pathways include the pentose phosphate pathway which generates pentose phosphates for ribonucleotides and NADPH; and the serine biosynthesis pathway which generates amino acids and initiates the one-carbon metabolism cycle [23]. Besides NADPH generation, one-carbon metabolism is also involved in the anabolic synthesis of amino acids, proteins, nucleotides and phospholipids, and has a role in the methylation reactions involved in post-translational modifications [24]. Additionally, during aerobic glycolysis, some glucose is diverted to glycerol-3 phosphate for fatty acid synthesis [21] and in the mitochondria, to the precursor, acetyl CoA for eventual cytosolic synthesis of lipids [22].

Apart from glucose metabolism, several other highly interconnected and multistep metabolic pathways and intermediates are involved in energy production and *de novo* synthesis of biomolecules. Other carbon fuels including glutamine, proline, serine, and fatty acids can ultimately feed into the TCA cycle to provide electron donors for the electron transport chain (ETC) and the generation of ATP [25]. Emerging evidence suggests a role for non-essential amino acids in tumor cell proliferation. For instance, arginine can promote tumor cell proliferation through nitric oxide synthesis. Additionally, the conversion of arginine to ornithine in the urea cycle, interconnects with the proline cycle leading to the generation of glutamate for the TCA cycle and glutamine synthesis [26]. Additionally, proline metabolism promotes cancer cell survival and energy production and regulates redox balance and biomass production [27]. The chemical energy of these fuels is harnessed by reducing electron carriers NAD+ and FAD to NADH and FADH2. These pathways eventually satisfy the three metabolic demands of cancer cells: (i) bioenergetics, (ii) macromolecular biosynthesis, and (iii) redox maintenance through $NADPH/NADP^+$ ratios. Additional pathways that regulate metabolic flux include MTOR, PI3K, AMPK, and autophagy [14].

However, there are multiple layers of complexity that should be accounted for when considering cancer metabolism. The heterogeneity of metabolism is multiple folds and can be attributed to (i) lineage-specific or selective expression alterations of metabolic transcripts that affect uptake, secretion, or other functions, (ii) genomic aberrations in metabolic genes such as mutations, deletions, amplification, and splicing events, (iii) epigenomic or non-genetic landscape changes, (iv) ATP generation affected by both cell type and the conditional context, (v) secondary metabolites of metabolism acting as tumor suppressors or oncogenes and (vi) stromal influences/tumor microenvironment.

'Metabolic' Dormancy and Related Biological Mechanisms

Altered tumor metabolism during dormancy need not consist entirely of adaptations that are driven to satisfy the bioenergetics demands of cell survival. Instead, such metabolic rewiring may also result in the development of specific dependencies that must be met to maintain cell survival [32–36]. For example, several tumor types are auxotrophic for one or more amino acids owing to deficiencies in a corresponding endogenous biosynthetic pathway. Particularly, some quiescent cells have a reliance on the import of amino acid(s), such as proline, from the extracellular matrix or serum [37] without which tumorigenesis ensues [38]. For instance, lymphoblastic leukemia and ovarian carcinomas depend on non-essential amino acid L-asparagine for survival [39]. Similarly, a large fraction of hepatocellular carcinomas, metastatic melanomas, and renal cell carcinomas are auxotrophic for L-arginine [40, 41]. The systemic depletion of such amino acids as a therapeutic strategy is of particular interest given the poor prognosis of these cancers and the difficulty in treating them with conventional chemotherapeutics.

Whereas tumor cells must maintain catabolic metabolism for the production of energy and anabolic metabolism for the synthesis of biomolecules required for rapid cell division, as mentioned above, dormant cells are relieved of this anabolic pressure and so presumably adopt a basal catabolic metabolism. Dormant tumor cells, thought to undergo a reversible cell cycle arrest in response to unfavorable conditions such as anti-neoplastic treatment, retain their ability to re-enter the proliferative cell cycle when conditions improve. This dormant phase is characterized by cell cycle arrest with 2N DNA, condensed chromosomes, reduced rRNA synthesis, decreased translation and decreased cell size [14]. Interestingly, non-neoplastic tissues including stem cells, eggs, spores and seeds respond similarly during conditions unfavorable to proliferation [28], accumulating DNA damage that is then repaired upon entry into cell cycle in the case of quiescent hematopoietic stem cells. In other accounts, such entry of hematopoietic stem cells into quiescence protects them from cytotoxic effects of chronic exposure to cytokines [29]. Survival of other types of tumors during stress-induced growth arrest, following therapy or growth factor withdrawal, depends on activation of stress and autophagy signaling pathways as well as survival signals (e.g. decorin) from the micro-environment (Fig. 3a) [30, 31]. Indeed, during dormancy, tumor cells are characterized by decreased rates of protein synthesis (via decreased MTOR activity) (Fig. 3c) and

Autophagy as a regulator of dormant tumour cell metabolism and survival

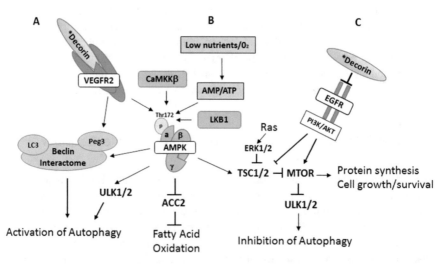

Fig. 3 Autophagy as a regulator of dormant tumour cell metabolism and survival. Treatment-induced dormant tumour cells lack adequate growth factors and nutrients and in a context-dependent manner, rely on compensatory signals from the extracellular matrix (ECM) and catabolic processes, such as autophagy, for energy and survival. (**a**) Decorin (DCN), a partial agonist of VEGFR2 induces autophagy through activation of AMPK and the association of the autophagy-initiation complex (Beclin interactome). (**b**) AMPK is activated by nutrient deprivation and low AMP/ATP ratios, as well as by LKB1 and CaMKKB which also induce autophagy. AMPK also inhibits ACC2 thus stimulating Fatty Acid Oxidation as a fuel source. (**c**) Decorin, binds EGFR and inhibits EGFR activation of MTOR, an inhibitor of ULK1 and autophagy

macromolecule synthesis [14]. To compensate for these deficiencies, dormant tumor cells may activate energy-sensing pathways including LBK1/AMPK-induced autophagy for the breakdown of macromolecules that allow them to reclaim energy and metabolites (Fig. 3b). The supply of these macromolecules can either be intracellular or come from a repertoire of matrix constituents (e.g. collagen network, decorin, laminin) [31]. Additionally, stress-response transcription factors (ATFs) and forkhead box subclass O3 (FoxO3) may enhance survival of dormant cells by activating PI3K/Rheb/ MTORC1 pathway in a context-dependent manner, thereby enabling these cells to adapt to their new environment [30].

Regulation of Metabolic Dormancy

The non-genetic component of metabolic dormancy attributed to stromal influences or metabolic intermediates cannot be underestimated as it can affect the final outcome of tumor fate. The hiding dormant niche can be exposed to differential vascularization that expose the tumors to varying spatial and temporal gradients of nutrients (energetics), oxygen (HIF1-induction in low concentrations), and pH (lactate secretion causing local acidification) [42, 43]. The alteration in metabolic pathways in dormancy is likely stimulated to adapt to such dynamic and energetically stressful conditions.

Both metabolic and proteostatic stress sensors are essential to adaptation to environmental stimuli such as therapy. These include transcription factors that regulate ER stress (i.e. IRE1α, PERK, ATF6, and XBP-1) or chaperones regulating the unfolded protein response (BiP, Grp78, HSP70 and -90) [44, 45]. Apart from these, metastasis-related transcription factors such as p53 loss [46], Sharp-1 [47], and NR2F1, regulated by the p38/ERK pathway, are also responsible for quiescence or cell cycle arrest of squamous carcinoma cells *in vivo* [48, 49]. P38 mitogen-activated protein kinase (MAPK) is one of the signaling pathways responsive to the stress stimuli and have been shown to be activated in quiescent tumor cells [49]. In hematopoietic stem cells, P38MAPK pathway restricts their cycling and promotes their entry into dormancy in the bone marrow niche [50].

Additionally, ROS and MTOR signaling pathways have also been associated with switching to a quiescence state in hematopoietic stem cells [51–53].

The Myc family of oncogenes are other transcriptional regulators of tumorigenesis, including genes involved cell growth and metabolism. However, depletion of Myc has varying effects in a context-dependent manner. For example, in mouse embryonic stem cells, inhibition of Myc decreases transcription of several genes leading to reversible cell cycle arrest and biosynthetic quiescence/dormancy [54]. Furthermore, highly quiescent dormant hematopoietic stem cells survive in a Myc-depleted environment whereas all other hematopoietic cells undergo apoptosis [55].

Apart from metabolic enzymes that act as tumor suppressors and oncogenes (e.g. succinate dehydrogenase, fumarate hydrogenase, isocitrate dehydrogenase among others), secondary metabolites and metabolic pathways in the context of tumor dormancy, one should also consider the two main regulatory axes of energy sensing: (i) PI3K/Akt/

mTORC and (ii) LBK1/AMPK/Autophagy. The well-characterized PI3K/Akt/MTOR pathway lies directly downstream of receptor tyrosine kinase (RTK) activation regulating glucose transporters, fatty acid synthesis, and growth. The AMP-activated protein kinase (AMPK), on the other hand, senses changes in the cellular ratio of AMP to ATP, allowing for adaptation to a metabolic stress. Under energetic stress, liver kinase B1 (LKB1), a tumor suppressor, regulated by AMPK, further regulates the signaling axis of metabolic control. As outlined in Fig. 3, these opposing pathways appear to be actively involved in regulating cellular dormancy or quiescence [56, 57].

The dormancy phase of cancer brings a renewed interest for the role of cellular metabolism and reappraises the notion that metabolic dormancy is a key feature of cancers that survive in their niche post therapy. It further proposes a renaissance for the potentials of metabolic targeting that have escaped scrutiny over the years.

Although we can expect that the metabolic rewiring during dormancy can revert back to that of normal proliferating cells, the dormant cells are presumably aberrantly driven by a combination of genetic lesions and non-genetic factors such as the tumor microenvironment [32]. For this reason and the inherent context-dependent heterogeneity of tumors, a single model of altered tumor metabolism does not describe the sum of metabolic changes that can support cellular quiescence. Thus, better understanding of metabolic dormancy can enable the development and optimization of therapeutic strategies that target tumor metabolism.

Technological, Biological, and Clinical Challenges to Study Metabolic Tumor Dormancy

The glycolytic activity of tumors is commonly exploited clinically by 18F-deoxyglucose positron emission tomography (FDG-PET). Radiolabeling of 18F-deoxyglucose helps in detecting tumors precisely by virtue of their enhanced ability to take up and metabolize glucose compared to normal tissue. However, the challenge with dormant tumors be it disseminated or residual, is that they are few in number, have minimal metabolic activities, and are often hidden from non-invasive detection (e.g. scanning technologies or blood stream circulation in the case of CTCs). Thus, the lack of drugs to target tumor dormancy and more specifically metabolic dormancy arises because of a lack of a mechanistic understanding of the dormancy phase and a lack of models for screening for new drugs that target this phase of cancer progression. Unfortunately, there are few cell lines that can exhibit a dormant phenotype in experimental mice partly because commonly used cell lines are selected for rapid metastatic ability. Hurst et al. has recently compiled recently compiled existing *in vitro* and *in vivo* models for dormancy for bone, lung, breast, ovarian, and pancreatic cancer [58]. We also wish to point to the existing models of patient-derived cell and tumor xenografts in prostate cancer [8, 9]. These *in vitro* and *in vivo* models can be therapeutically treated to enter a therapy-induced dormancy phase and so offer an improved alternative for the study of metabolic dormancy [1, 9] and understanding the inherent heterogeneous diversity of different cancer types. These models can be used for biochemical, transcriptomic, and metabolomics studies, not entirely dissimilar to approaches used for cancer stem cell investigations [59–63]. These studies are expected to refine cancer-specific dormant cell markers that allow soring of cells to a high purity for functional *in vitro* assays or *in vivo* re-transplantations. Beyond these studies, suitable models for tumor metabolism *in vivo* such that it mimics the physiological conditions of the microenvironment are extremely rare [64]. The metabolic dependencies and liabilities within a given tumor cell should then ideally guide the utilization of specific radiolabeling and technology requirements. This is further exacerbated by the challenges involved in designing clinical trials that address tumor and cellular dormancy. Although these reasons hamper the development of new approaches to *in vivo* metabolic analyses, there are several breast cancer clinical trials designed for studying breast cancer progression following adjuvant treatments, i.e. TEACH [64, 65], HERA trial [66], or metastatic prostate cancer progression in NCT00309985 trial [67]. Thus, recognition of tumor dormancy complexity aided by the progress of various "omics"-based strategies ideally leads to the continued exploitation and integration of imaging technologies.

Premise of Therapeutic Targeting of Metabolic Dormancy

Given that metabolic reprogramming in cancers is widely recognized, therapeutic targeting of this rewiring has garnered significant attention and investigation. However, there remains a vast disconnect between identification of dormant tumors and the design of appropriate clinical trials. Targeting of tumor dormancy, therefore, remains an elusive field of research. This is expected for the difficulty of detecting and targeting this phase of cancer. Some of the first-line chemotherapeutic agents, such as nucleoside analogues and antimetabolites that target the direct inhibition of enzymes used in DNA synthesis, are no longer feasible for dormancy. Other therapeutic opportunities explored for cancers, small-molecule inhibition of key enzymes involved in metabolic pathways such as glycolysis and fatty acid synthesis, offer limited potential. These strategies are equally unspecific and irrelevant in the context of dormancy. Therefore, we need to rethink the development of strategies that target this 'therapeutic window' of cancer. One crucial consideration that remains common in the development of anticancer therapeutics irrespective of dormancy is to the extent to which a given drug can achieve its intended mechanism of action without additionally exerting unacceptable toxicities for normal cells. This is especially relevant as any targeting strategy for the dormancy phase will be aimed either for long-term maintenance of dormancy without stimulating a malignant evolution (let the sleeping dogs lie) or killing the cells as they sleep [64].

Conclusions

The collection of advances made in our understanding of tumor metabolism in recent years is not sufficient for targeting metabolically dormant cancer cells. Therefore, a better understanding of the diversity of mechanistic adaptations and context-dependent determinants that can drive metabolic rewiring of dormant cancer cells is direly required. As our understanding of dormant tumor metabolism continues to evolve by advances in analytical technologies and animal models, we can progress in capitalizing upon the exploitation of their atypical metabolic features. Finally, distinguishing the interplay between genetic and microenvironmental elements of tumor dormancy can serve as critical factors in determining therapeutic targets that enable maximal drug efficacy and minimal deleterious effects on normal cells.

Financial Support This work was supported by the Canadian Institutes of Health Research (Y.W.), BC Cancer Foundation Mesothelioma Research Fund/Mitacs Accelerate Postdoctoral Fellowship Fund (N.N., Y.W., C.C.C.), and the Terry Fox New Frontiers Program on Prostate Cancer Progression (C.C.C., Y.W.).

Conflicts of Interest The authors confirm that there are no conflicts of interest.

References

1. Aguirre-Ghiso JA (2007) Models, mechanisms and clinical evidence for cancer dormancy. Nat Rev Cancer 7(11):834–846. PubMed PMID: PMC2519109
2. Friedlander TW, Fong L (2014) The end of the beginning: circulating tumor cells as a biomarker in castration-resistant prostate cancer. J Clin Oncol 32(11):1104–1106. PubMed PMID: 24616311
3. Paget S (1889) The distribution of secondary growths in cancer of the breast. The Lancet. 133(3421):571–573
4. Hinck L (2011) Tumor suppressors: heroes and villains? J Mammary Gland Biol Neoplasia 16(3):169–171. PubMed PMID: PMC4105358
5. Jäger W, Xue H, Hayashi T, Janssen C, Awrey S, Wyatt AW et al (2015) Patient-derived bladder cancer xenografts in the preclinical development of novel targeted therapies. Oncotarget 6(25):21522–21532
6. Eirew P, Steif A, Khattra J, Ha G, Yap D, Farahani H et al (2015) Dynamics of genomic clones in breast cancer patient xenografts at single-cell resolution. Nature 518(7539):422–426
7. Choi SYC, Lin D, Gout PW, Collins CC, Xu Y, Wang Y (2014) Lessons from patient-derived xenografts for better in vitro modeling of human cancer. Adv Drug Deliv Rev 79–80:222–237
8. Lin D, Xue H, Wang Y, Wu R, Watahiki A, Dong X et al (2014) Next generation patient-derived prostate cancer xenograft models. Asian J Androl 16(3):407–412
9. Lin D, Wyatt AW, Xue H, Wang Y, Dong X, Haegert A et al (2014) High fidelity patient-derived xenografts for accelerating prostate cancer discovery and drug development. Cancer Res 74(4):1272–1283
10. Radzikowski J (2013) Resistance of dormant stages of planktonic invertebrates to adverse environmental conditions. J Plankton Res 35(4):707–723
11. Archuleta RJ, Yvonne Hoppes P, Primm TP (2005) Mycobacterium Avium enters a state of metabolic dormancy in response to starvation. Tuberculosis 85(3):147–158
12. Chubukov V, Sauer U (2014) Environmental dependence of stationary-phase metabolism in Bacillus Subtilis and Escherichia coli. Appl Environ Microbiol 80(9):2901–2909
13. Shimizu K (2014) Regulation Systems of Bacteria such as Escherichia coli in response to nutrient limitation and environmental stresses. Metabolites 4(1):1. doi:10.3390/metabo4010001
14. Valcourt JR, Lemons JMS, Haley EM, Kojima M, Demuren OO, Coller HA (2012) Staying alive. Cell Cycle 11(9):1680–1696
15. van der Toom EE, Verdone JE, Pienta KJ (2016) Disseminated tumor cells and dormancy in prostate cancer metastasis. Curr Opin Biotechnol 40:9–15

16. Lam H-M, Vessella RL, Morrissey C (2014) The role of the microenvironment—dormant prostate disseminated tumor cells in the bone marrow. Drug Discov Today Technol 11:41–47. PubMed PMID: PMC4412595
17. Shiozawa Y, Eber MR, Berry JE, Taichman RS (2015) Bone marrow as a metastatic niche for disseminated tumor cells from solid tumors. BoneKEy Rep 4:689
18. Amoêdo Nívea D, Valencia Juan P, Rodrigues Mariana F, Galina A, Rumjanek FD (2013) How does the metabolism of tumour cells differ from that of normal cells. Biosci Rep 33(6):e00080. PubMed PMID: PMC3828821
19. Cantor JR, Sabatini DM (2012) Cancer cell metabolism: one hallmark, many faces. Cancer Discov 2(10):881–898
20. Warburg O (1956) On the origin of cancer cells. Science 123(3191):309–314
21. Hay N (2016) Reprogramming glucose metabolism in cancer: can it be exploited for cancer therapy? Nat Rev Cancer 16(10):635–649
22. Vander Heiden MG, Cantley LC, Thompson CB (2009) Understanding the Warburg effect: the metabolic requirements of cell proliferation. Science 324(5930):1029–1033
23. Mattaini KR, Sullivan MR, Vander Heiden MG (2016) The importance of serine metabolism in cancer. J Cell Biol 214(3):249–257
24. Locasale JW (2013) Serine, glycine and one-carbon units: cancer metabolism in full circle. Nat Rev Cancer 13(8):572–583
25. Phang JM, Liu W, Hancock CN, Fischer JW (2015) Proline metabolism and cancer: emerging links to glutamine and collagen. Curr Opin Clin Nutr Metab Care 18(1):71–77. PubMed PMID: 00075197-201501000-00012
26. Olivares O, Däbritz JHM, King A, Gottlieb E, Halsey C (2015) Research into cancer metabolomics: towards a clinical metamorphosis. Semin Cell Dev Biol 43:52–64
27. Phang JM, Liu W, Hancock C (2013) Bridging epigenetics and metabolism: role of nonessential amino acids. Epigenetics 8(3):231–236. PubMed PMID: PMC3669115
28. Beerman I, Seita J, Inlay Matthew A, Weissman Irving L, Rossi DJ (2014) Quiescent hematopoietic stem cells accumulate DNA damage during aging that is repaired upon entry into cell cycle. Cell Stem Cell 15(1):37–50
29. Pietras EM, Lakshminarasimhan R, Techner J-M, Fong S, Flach J, Binnewies M et al (2014) Re-entry into quiescence protects hematopoietic stem cells from the killing effect of chronic exposure to type I interferons. J Exp Med 211(2):245–262
30. Sosa MS, Bragado P, Debnath J, Aguirre-Ghiso JA (2013) Regulation of tumor cell dormancy by tissue microenvironments and autophagy. Adv Exp Med Biol 734:73–89. PubMed PMID: PMC3651695
31. Neill T, Schaefer L, Iozzo RV (2014) Instructive roles of extracellular matrix on autophagy. Am J Pathol 184(8):2146–2153
32. Ito K, Suda T (2014) Metabolic requirements for the maintenance of self-renewing stem cells. Nat Rev Mol Cell Biol 15(4):243–256
33. Ward PS, Thompson CB (2012) Signaling in control of cell growth and metabolism. Cold Spring Harbor Perspect Biol 4(7):a006783. PubMed PMID: PMC3385956
34. Krall AS, Xu S, Graeber TG, Braas D, Christofk HR (2016) Asparagine promotes cancer cell proliferation through use as an amino acid exchange factor. Nat Commun 7:11457
35. Yang M, Vousden KH (2016) Serine and one-carbon metabolism in cancer. Nat Rev Cancer 16(10):650–662
36. Ducker Gregory S, Rabinowitz JD (2017) One-carbon metabolism in health and disease. Cell Metab 25(1):27–42
37. Saqcena M, Menon D, Patel D, Mukhopadhyay S, Chow V, Foster DA (2013) Amino acids and mtor mediate distinct metabolic checkpoints in mammalian G1 cell cycle. PLoS One 8(8):e74157. PubMed PMID: PMC3747087
38. Sahu N, Dela Cruz D, Gao M, Sandoval W, Haverty Peter M, Liu J et al (2016) Proline starvation induces unresolved ER stress and hinders mTORC1-dependent tumorigenesis. Cell Metab 24(5):753–761
39. Tsun Z-Y, Possemato R (2015) Amino acid management in cancer. Semin Cell Dev Biol 43:22–32. PubMed PMID: PMC4800996

40. Phillips MM, Sheaff MT, Szlosarek PW (2013) Targeting arginine-dependent cancers with arginine-degrading enzymes: opportunities and challenges. Cancer Res Treat 45(4):251–262
41. Patil MD, Bhaumik J, Babykutty S, Banerjee UC, Fukumura D (2016) Arginine dependence of tumor cells: targeting a chink in cancer/'s armor. Oncogene 35(38):4957–4972
42. Chiang C-H, Chang M-Y, Hsu J-J, Chiu T-H, Lee K-F, Ts-Ta H et al (1999) Tumor vascular pattern and blood flow impedance in the differential diagnosis of leiomyoma and adenomyosis by color doppler sonography. J Assist Reprod Genet 16(5):268–275. PubMed PMID: PMC3455709
43. Antonescu C (2014) Malignant vascular tumors—an update. Mod Pathol 27(S1):S30–SS8
44. Urra H, Dufey E, Avril T, Chevet E, Hetz C (2016) Endoplasmic reticulum stress and the hallmarks of cancer. Trends Cancer 2(5):252–262
45. Tsai YC, Weissman AM (2010) The unfolded protein response, degradation from the endoplasmic reticulum, and cancer. Genes Cancer 1(7):764–778. PubMed PMID: PMC3039444
46. Powell E, Piwnica-Worms D, Piwnica-Worms H (2014) Contribution of p53 to metastasis. Cancer Discov 4(4):405–414
47. Montagner M, Enzo E, Forcato M, Zanconato F, Parenti A, Rampazzo E et al (2012) SHARP1 suppresses breast cancer metastasis by promoting degradation of hypoxia-inducible factors. Nature 487(7407):380–384
48. Adam AP, George A, Schewe D, Bragado P, Iglesias BV, Ranganathan AC et al (2009) Computational identification of a p38^{SAPK}-regulated transcription factor network required for tumor cell quiescence. Cancer Res 69(14):5664
49. Aguirre-Ghiso JA, Estrada Y, Liu D, Ossowski L (2003) ERK-MAPK activity as a determinant of tumor growth and dormancy; regulation by p38-SAPK. Cancer Res 63(7):1684
50. Tesio M, Tang Y, Müdder K, Saini M, von Paleske L, Macintyre E et al (2015) Hematopoietic stem cell quiescence and function are controlled by the CYLD–TRAF2–p38MAPK pathway. J Exp Med 212(4):525
51. Ludin A, Gur-Cohen S, Golan K, Kaufmann KB, Itkin T, Medaglia C et al (2014) Reactive oxygen species regulate hematopoietic stem cell self-renewal, migration and development, as well as their bone marrow microenvironment. Antioxid Redox Signal 21(11):1605–1619. PubMed PMID: PMC4175025
52. Bigarella CL, Liang R, Ghaffari S (2014) Stem cells and the impact of ROS signaling. Development 141(22):4206–4218
53. Huang J, Nguyen-McCarty M, Hexner EO, Danet-Desnoyers G, Klein PS (2012) Maintenance of hematopoietic stem cells through regulation of Wnt and mTOR pathways. Nat Med 18(12):1778–1785
54. Scognamiglio R, Cabezas-Wallscheid N, Thier Marc C, Altamura S, Reyes A, Prendergast Áine M et al (2016) Myc depletion induces a pluripotent dormant state mimicking diapause. Cell 164(4):668–680
55. Laurenti E, Wilson A, Trumpp A (2009) Myc's other life: stem cells and beyond. Curr Opin Cell Biol 21(6):844–854
56. Yeh AC, Ramaswamy S (2015) Mechanisms of cancer cell dormancy—another hallmark of cancer? Cancer Res 75(23):5014–5022
57. Rodgers JT, King KY, Brett JO, Cromie MJ, Charville GW, Maguire KK et al (2014) mTORC1 controls the adaptive transition of quiescent stem cells from G0 to GAlert. Nature 510(7505):393–396
58. Hurst RE, Bastian A, Bailey-Downs L, Ihnat MA (2016) Targeting dormant micrometastases: rationale, evidence to date and clinical implications. Ther Adv Med Oncol 8(2):126–137. PubMed PMID: PMC4753353
59. Won EJ, Kim H-R, Park R-Y, Choi S-Y, Shin JH, Suh S-P et al (2015) Direct confirmation of quiescence of CD34+CD38- leukemia stem cell populations using single cell culture, their molecular signature and clinicopathological implications. BMC Cancer 15:217. PubMed PMID: PMC4391681

60. Chen W, Dong J, Haiech J, Kilhoffer M-C, Zeniou M (2016) Cancer stem cell quiescence and plasticity as major challenges in cancer therapy. Stem Cells Int 2016:1740936. PubMed PMID: PMC4932171
61. Buczacki S, Davies RJ, Winton DJ (2011) Stem cells, quiescence and rectal carcinoma: an unexplored relationship and potential therapeutic target. Br J Cancer 105(9):1253–1259. PubMed PMID: PMC3241542
62. Suresh R, Ali S, Ahmad A, Philip PA, Sarkar FH (2016) The role of cancer stem cells in recurrent and drug-resistant lung cancer. In: Ahmad A, Gadgeel SM (eds) Lung cancer and personalized medicine: novel therapies and clinical management. Springer, Cham, pp 57–74
63. Han L, Shi S, Gong T, Zhang Z, Sun X (2013) Cancer stem cells: therapeutic implications and perspectives in cancer therapy. Acta Pharm Sin B 3(2):65–75
64. Goss PE, Chambers AF (2010) Does tumour dormancy offer a therapeutic target? Nat Rev Cancer 10(12):871–877
65. Loi S, Dafni U, Karlis D et al (2016) Effects of estrogen receptor and human epidermal growth factor receptor-2 levels on the efficacy of trastuzumab: a secondary analysis of the hera trial. JAMA Oncol 2(8):1040–1047
66. Piccart-Gebhart MJ, Procter M, Leyland-Jones B, Goldhirsch A, Untch M, Smith I et al (2005) Trastuzumab after adjuvant chemotherapy in HER2-positive breast cancer. N Engl J Med 353(16):1659–1672. PubMed PMID: 16236737
67. Sweeney CJ, Chen Y-H, Carducci M, Liu G, Jarrard DF, Eisenberger M et al (2015) Chemohormonal therapy in metastatic hormone-sensitive prostate cancer. N Engl J Med 373(8):737–746. PubMed PMID: 26244877

Tumor Dormancy, Angiogenesis and Metronomic Chemotherapy

Gianfranco Natale and Guido Bocci

Abstract Angiogenic dormancy can be defined as the condition in which cancer cell proliferation is counterbalanced by apoptosis owing to poor vascularization. Indeed, the lack of tumor angiogenesis impedes tumor mass expansion beyond a microscopic size, resulting in an asymptomatic and non-metastatic state. Thus, the tumor angiogenic switch is essential to promote fast-growing and expansion of tumor masses and to develop the metastatic process. In the avascular tumor lesion, angiogenesis process results blocked from the equilibrium between pro- and anti-angiogenic factors, such as vascular endothelial growth factor (VEGF) and thrombospondin-1 (TSP-1), respectively. The angiogenic switch of non-dormant tumors mainly depends on the disruption of the balance in the tumor microenvironment between anti-angiogenic and pro-angiogenic factors, in favor of the latter. Moreover, this tumors activate and recruit the circulating endothelial progenitors (CEPs) that facilitate the shift toward the generation of new blood vessels. Metronomic chemotherapy—a regular administration of drug doses able to maintain low but active concentrations of chemotherapeutic drugs during prolonged periods of time—is a promising therapeutic approach that can induce or re-induce the angiogenic tumor dormancy. Metronomic chemotherapy upregulates TSP-1 and decreases pro-angiogenic factors such as VEGF, and suppresses the proangiogenic cells such as CEPs both in adjuvant setting or in the treatment of metastatic disease. In this perspective, metronomic chemotherapy may be able to play a main role in the modulation of the angiogenic tumor dormancy, but further preclinical and clinical studies are needed to better investigate this particular aspect of this interesting therapeutic tool.

Keywords Tumor dormancy • Angiogenesis • Metronomic chemotherapy • Thrombospondin-1 • Vascular endothelial growth factor • Circulating endothelial progenitor

G. Natale, M.D.
Dipartimento di Ricerca Traslazionale e delle Nuove Tecnologie in Medicina e Chirurgia, and Museo di Anatomia Umana "Filippo Civinini", Università di Pisa, Pisa, Italy

G. Bocci, M.D., Ph.D. (✉)
Dipartimento di Medicina Clinica e Sperimentale, Università di Pisa,
Scuola Medica – Via Roma 55, 56126 Pisa, Italy
e-mail: guido.bocci@med.unipi.it

© Springer International Publishing AG 2017
Y. Wang, F. Crea (eds.), *Tumor Dormancy and Recurrence*, Cancer Drug Discovery and Development, DOI 10.1007/978-3-319-59242-8_3

Introduction

The concept of tumor dormancy refers to the presence of asymptomatic and temporarily non-invasive cancer cells which are diagnostically undetected for months or decades. Indeed, autopsies of several people who did not die for tumors revealed the accidental presence of non-expanding microscopic primary cancer and the occurrence of these non-invasive dormant cells can be considered "normal" in healthy subjects [1]. Nevertheless, this condition of occult cancer can represent the early stage of tumor development, but it can also account for tumor recurrence after a successful treatment, as well as micro-metastases. Accordingly, cancer progression can be regarded as a multistep process. Both experimental and clinical studies suggest that cancer cell dissemination occur at very early stages of tumor growth and that these disseminated cells can remain dormant for a long time. The phenomenon of metastatic tumor dormancy is on the basis of tumor metastasis which can occur also several years after an apparently effective therapy. Then, tumor dormancy is clinically relevant in both primary and secondary tumors, which arise from residual disseminated cancer cells. However, the peculiar features of tumor dormancy impede to have appropriate experimental models and clinical accessibility and the problem remains poorly investigated [2–4].

It is important to distinguish between quiescent solitary cells (tumor cell dormancy) and small-sized asymptomatic cancerous lesions (tumor dormancy). Indeed, these two types of dormancy represent completely distinct conditions that significantly differ in their characteristics and underlying regulatory mechanisms [3].

It is particularly noteworthy to identify those factors that are able either to maintain cancer cells in an occult state or to promote the escape from dormancy. Taking into account that preventing screening tests are unable to reveal such undetectable abnormal solitary cells, the knowledge of tumor dormancy pathophysiology is essential to understand cancer development and to design therapeutic strategies. Tumor dormancy would involve quiescence, consisting of reversible cell cycle arrest. However, some tumor cells seem to be also able to reverse senescence, consisting of permanent cell cycle arrest, and a combination of both mechanisms might lead to tumor dormancy [4–6].

The complex interactions occurring in the tumor microenvironment, in particular the relationship of the cancer cell with the extracellular matrix and other normal cell types (e.g., endothelial cells, fibroblast), appear determinant in contrasting tumor growth. The expression of some receptors, including urokinase and epidermal growth factor (EGF) receptors, has been associated to the regulation of the quiescence-based dormancy of tumors [7, 8]. Considering the ability of different organs to support disseminated tumor cells growth, microenvironments have been classified as dormancy-permissive or dormancy-restrictive and this distinction might account for the different incidence of metastases and disseminated tumor cells in the same organ ("seed and soil" theory) [9, 10].

The immune surveillance plays a pivotal role in suppressing cancer growth and both cellular and humoral responses are needed to maintain the occult state of cancer mass [11]. However, the inflammatory state that associates to the release of cytokines during some immune reactions can trigger angiogenesis-mediated escape from dormancy [12].

Specific changes in cytoskeleton architecture, involving fibronectin production and activation of integrin β-1 signalling pathway, may be associated to the pattern of the dormant cell [13].

Other factors that facilitate the permanence of the tumor in a dormant state include the hormonal withdrawal and the inhibition of angiogenesis [3, 14, 15]. Apart from adjuvant chemotherapy strategies, various dietary components, in terms of food intake, energy balance and physical activity, might also influence cancer cells and their microenvironment. Indeed, several dietary phytochemicals can affect the behavior and gene expression patterns of both tumor cells and host tissues [16].

The Role of Angiogenesis in Tumor Dormancy

Angiogenesis is a biologic process consisting in the formation of new capillaries from pre-existing blood vessels [17]. This process occurs in several physiological conditions, including embryogenesis, ovulation, wound healing and repair. However, it can be also observed in pathological conditions, such as arthritis, diabetic retinopathy, endometriosis and tumors. The growth of solid tumors includes an avascular and a subsequent vascular phase. Most tumors seem to begin as small sized and non-angiogenic cellular aggregates which cannot grow until vascular network is established. Indeed, an important mechanism behind tumor dormancy is the ability of cancer cells to induce angiogenesis. In solid tumors the transition from the avascular to the vascular phase is critical for the proliferation of cancer cells *in situ* and at distant sites, as metastases. In this respect, tumor growth is thought to be angiogenesis-dependent and the inhibitors of angiogenesis have been then proposed as anticancer therapy [18, 19].

Not surprisingly, a pivotal mechanism behind tumor dormancy is represented by the ability of tumor cells to induce angiogenesis and, more importantly, to realize successfully and correctly the complete process of new blood vessel formation. Indeed, failure in one or more of the angiogenic steps leads to dormancy [3].

Tumor dormancy may be referred to a single cancer cell (tumor cell dormancy) which lies in cell cycle arrest (G0-G1 arrest), or to active proliferating tumor cells (tumor mass dormancy) whose growth is significantly limited by efficient immune surveillance, or insufficient blood supply (angiogenic dormancy), leading to dynamic equilibrium between cell proliferation and apoptotic death. In fact, dormant tumor cells are generally considered in an arrested state, but a debate exists whether micrometastatic disease consists in a balance of cell proliferation and death that only appears as an arrested state [6, 10].

Aguirre-Ghiso [6] just defined angiogenic dormancy the condition in which cancer cell proliferation is counterbalanced by apoptosis owing to poor vascularization. As a consequence, the cancer cells are unable to grow. Then, malignant properties of cancer cells are not enough to develop a tumor that becomes lethal: a cancer without disease! Tumor angiogenesis is strictly necessary to promote fast-growing and expansion. The lack of tumor angiogenesis impedes tumor mass expansion beyond a microscopic size, resulting in an asymptomatic and non-metastatic state [20].

The normal angiogenesis results from the equilibrium between pro- and anti-angiogenic factors. The first pro-angiogenic factor, named tumor angiogenic factor (TAF), was hypothesized 45 years ago by Judah Folkman [21], who also suggested that tumor growth strongly depends on angiogenesis and proposed anti-angiogenic therapy as a new approach to treat cancer disease [22]. In subsequent years, other receptor-mediated agents activating and regulating angiogenesis were identified, among which fibroblast growth factors 1 and 2 (FGF-1 and 2) [23], the most important vascular endothelial growth factor (VEGF) family (VEGF A to D) [17], placenta growth factor (PLGF) [24], platelet-derived growth factors (PDGFs), insulin-like growth factors (IGFs), angiopoietin 1, EGF, hepatocyte growth factor (HGF), hypoxia-inducible factor-1 α and β (HIF-1 α and β), transforming growth factor-α and β (TGF-α and β), tumor necrosis factor-α (TNF-α), interleukins (IL)-1 β, 3, 6, 8, neuropilin 1 and 2, angiogenin, adrenomedullin, stromal cell-derived factor-1 (SDF-1) [18, 25, 26].

Apart from hypoxia, other environmental stressors are able to induce the expression of pro-angiogenic factors, including glucose deprivation, accumulation of reactive oxygen species (ROS), cellular acidosis or iron deficiency, or the activation of oncogenes, such as Ras [27] and Myc, or the loss of the function of tumor suppressor genes [3].

Dormant cancer cells appear to undergo a stable genetic reprogramming process during their escape towards the fast-growing phenotype and this would occur during the angiogenic switch: progress from non-angiogenic to angiogenic phenotype, with recruitment of new blood vessels. This condition is considered an early marker of neoplastic transformation. Although dysfunctional, with irregular shape and architecture, tumor blood vessels are essential for the growth of malignant cancer cells. An important concept is that the acquisition of angiogenic capacity is required a long time before the emergence of an invasive malignancy [3].

Human tumors contain cancer cell subpopulations with different angiogenic potential. In a human liposarcoma cell line (SW-872), three different clone patterns of growth have been isolated and observed: highly angiogenic clones with rapid tumor growth; weakly angiogenic clones with slow tumor growth; non-angiogenic clones corresponding to vital but dormant tumors and also named "non-tumorigenic" or "no-take". This concept has been also explored in animal models of tumor dormancy, especially by inoculating human cancer cells in immunocompromised mice [20, 28].

Environmental hypoxia in cancer cell proliferation appears to be a crucial factor inducing angiogenic switch, this expression indicating the transition from the non-angiogenic to the angiogenic tumor phenotype, with subsequent disease progression. When a small-sized tumor mass attempts to grow, central cancer cells remain too distant from normal surrounding blood vessels to benefit of oxygen diffusion and tend to necrosis. This hypoxic condition might trigger compensatory mechanisms in suffering cells, with an increased expression and activation of the transcription factor HIF-1 pathway or HIF-1-independent pathways, as well. Subsequently, other pro-angiogenic factors are recruited, including VEGF, PDGF and nitric oxide (NO) synthase. The angiogenic switch would depend on the disruption of the normal equilibrium in the microenvironment between anti-angiogenic and pro-angiogenic factors, in favor of the latter. The initial step is represented by hyperemic reaction at the periphery of the tumor, due to vasodilation, followed by a process of angiogenesis. A transient angiogenic switch delivered by factors of the tumor microenvironment can also convey tumorigenic properties to cancer cells [12, 14, 29].

In particular, the switch of dormant cancer cells was associated with downregulation of the angiogenesis inhibitor thrombospondin-1 (TSP-1) and decreased sensitivity to angiostatin. Cancer cell secretion and intracellular levels of TSP-1 in non-angiogenic and angiogenic tumor cell populations isolated from the human breast cancer cell line MDAMB-436 were compared, indicating that angiogenic cancer cells contain significantly lower levels of TSP-1 than non-angiogenic tumor cells and secretion of TSP-1 from non-angiogenic tumor cells was 20-fold higher than angiogenic cells. The decrease in TSP-1 levels seems to be mediated by phosphatidylinositol 3-kinase (PI3K) [30, 31].

It was shown that in the endothelium the expression of the angiogenesis inducers epoxyeicosatrienoic acids (EETs) stimulated escape from tumor dormancy in mice. In line with this, EETs stimulated metastasis of various xenograft tumors, including Lewis lung carcinomas (LLC) and B16-F10 melanomas [32].

The Notch signaling pathway is largely used by endothelial cells to coordinate cellular activities during the blood vessel formation that occurs in angiogenesis. Then, not surprisingly, an interactive cross-talk between cancer and endothelial cells has been shown to favor the escape of tumors from dormancy, this transition being mediated by the Notch ligand Dll4 on endothelial cells and Notch 3 signaling in tumor cells, promoting a tumorigenic phenotype. In agreement with this, Notch 3 levels are low in dormant tumors. These data provide a novel angiogenesis-driven mechanism involving the Notch pathway in controlling tumor dormancy. Metabolic features also participate in the regulation of tumor dormancy. The activity of the LKB1/AMPK system, deputed to monitor cellular ATP levels, is enhanced by anti-VEGF therapy, leading to glucose depletion and reduction of ATP levels, with tumor regression [10, 33, 34].

It was reported that local traumas, injuries, wounds, burns and surgery can cause a permissive microenvironmental niche for tumor growth. These conditions are unlike to induce the onset of malignant cells, rather they promote the escape from tumor dormancy. The occurrence of an inflammatory state and the ability to attract circulating cancer cells or to mobilize circulating endothelial progenitors (CEPs), with an increase in VEGF plasma levels, might explain such a transition to a non-dormant state [7, 14].

Apart from cancer cells themselves and local stromal microenvironment, distant bone marrow cells, once recruited into tumor masses, also participate to the induction of the angiogenic switch. The stromal cells that surround tumor masses mainly include fibroblasts, lymphocytes, neutrophils, macrophages and mast cells, which communicate through intercellular signalling pathways, mediated by surface adhesion molecules, cytokines and their receptors. Paradoxically, infiltrating cells of the immune system are important constituents of tumors and can represent a fundamental source of growth stimulatory signals. Although at a different extent and with data still debated, several bone marrow-derived cell (BMDC) types have been implicated in the escape from tumor dormancy, as well as in the metastatic dissemination. These cells include endothelial progenitor cells, Tie-2 expressing monocytes, the heterogeneous family of immature myeloid cells, hemangiocytes, M1 and M2 tumor associated macrophages, dendritic cells, and mast cells. As in other pathophysiologic conditions such as healing, infection, inflammation or ischemia, several cytokines and chemokines would be released by cancer cells to recruit a large body of BMDC types which contribute to the angiogenic switch. In this respect, inflammation is regarded as a strong promoter for angiogenic switch, and also circulating platelets have been implicated in the transport and dissemination of such pro-angiogenic factor [3, 7, 35]. These data suggest that a lot of angiogenic factors are required to trigger tumor angiogenesis. On this basis, Indraccolo et al. [36] proposed the "spike hypothesis", according to which a transient but consistent supply of angiogenic factors is able to promote the angiogenic switch.

The exosomes released by cancer cells contain soluble cytokines, growth factors, integrins, mRNA and microRNA which are able to reprogram bone marrow progenitor cells with pro-angiogenic and pro-metastatic activity [37]. In particular, exosomes released by renal carcinoma cells were able to activate an angiogenic phenotype in normal endothelial cells *in vitro* and tumor cell colonization of the lung and angiogenesis *in vivo* [38].

Some data indicate that certain tumors are able to transform bone marrow cells into pro-tumorigenic even prior to their mobilization into the circulation. This process through which humoral signals released from certain tumors stimulate bone marrow cells, which are mobilized into the circulation and subsequently induce the growth of otherwise dormant cancer cells residing at distant anatomical sites, is defined systemic instigation. Certain breast tumors (instigators) release the cytokine osteopontin (OPN) into the circulation and tumor-derived OPN programs hematopoietic progenitor cells to adopt a pro-tumorigenic state, in part, by inducing their over-expression of the secreted glycoprotein, granulin (GRN) [39].

Autophagy is a highly conserved self-degradative mechanism that plays an important role in removing dysfunctional cellular components and takes part in several physiopathological processes, including starvation, infections, programmed cell death, repair and degenerative mechanisms. Its role in cancer is dual. From one hand, it promotes survival of cancer cells, and from the other hand, it behaves as a tumor suppressor. In this respect, autophagy seems to favour tumor dormancy by inducing growth arrest with consequent prevention of programmed cell death, according to the dormant stem-like state of cancer cells. Accordingly, stimulation of autophagy induces quiescence and growth arrest in cancer cells, whereas inhibition of autophagy causes rapid cell death. In M2 tumor associated macrophages and fibroblasts, autophagy seems to promote pro-invasive, pro-angiogenic and pro-metastatic phenotype [37].

Considering that the transition from dormant to fast-growing tumor is angiogenesis-dependent and requires a stable transcriptional reprogramming, this phenomenon has been also evaluated by genome analysis. Cancer cells expressing microRNA cluster 126 (miR-126) have been shown to reduce the recruitment of endothelial cells to the tumor site by blocking GAS6/MER signaling [40]. It was

Table 1 Definition of non-angiogenic/dormant tumors, modified from [14, 20]

1. Tumors are unable to induce angiogenic activity, by avoiding existing blood vessels in the local stroma and/or relative absence of intratumoral microvessels
2. Tumors remain harmless to the host until they switch to the angiogenic phenotype
3. Tumors express equal or more anti-angiogenic (i.e., TSP-1) than pro-angiogenic (i.e., VEGF, bFGF) proteins
4. Tumors grow *in vivo* to ~1 mm in diameter or less, at which time further expansion ceases
5. Tumors are only visible with a hand lens or a dissecting microscope (5–10x magnification)
6. Tumors are white or transparent by gross examination
7. Tumors are unable to spontaneously metastasize from the microscopic dormant state
8. Tumors show active cell proliferation and apoptosis *in vivo* and remain metabolically active during the dormancy period
9. Human tumors are heterogeneous and contain both non-angiogenic and angiogenic cells: In dormant tumors the non-angiogenic promoting cells are prevalent

Table 2 Definition of angiogenic/non-dormant tumors, modified from [14, 20]

1. Tumors are able to induce angiogenic activity, by recruiting blood vessels from the surrounding stroma and/or forming new blood vessels within the tumor tissue
2. Tumors are lethal to the host if not treated
3. Tumors express significantly more pro-angiogenic than anti-angiogenic proteins
4. Tumors grow along an exponential curve until they kill the host
5. Tumors are visible and easily detectable based on their macroscopic size
6. Tumors appear red by gross examination
7. Tumors can spontaneously metastasize to various organs
8. Tumors show very active cell proliferation and a low grade of apoptosis *in vivo* during the growth period
9. Human tumors are heterogeneous and contain both non-angiogenic and angiogenic cells: In non-dormant tumors the angiogenic promoting cells are prevalent

also observed that suppression of the heat shock protein (HSP) 27 associates the non-angiogenic pattern with the inhibition of endothelial cell proliferation leading to long-term dormancy in human breast cancer [41]. Almog et al., [42] evaluated 19 microRNAs dealing with the phenotypic switch to fast-growth of four human dormant tumors: breast carcinoma, glioblastoma, osteosarcoma, and liposarcoma. Loss of expression of dormancy-associated microRNAs was the prevailing regulation pattern correlating with the switch of dormant tumors to fast-growth. Reconstitution of a single dormant microRNA led to phenotypic reversal of fast-growing angiogenic tumors towards long-lasting tumor dormancy. Furthermore, transcriptional reprogramming of tumors by means of dormant microRNAs over-expression led to down-regulation of pro-angiogenic factors, such as bFGF and TGF-α. Anti-angiogenic and dormancy promoting pathways such as EphA5 and angiomotin were up-regulated in dormant microRNA over-expressing tumors [42].

Taking into account the above-mentioned features of angiogenesis in tumor dormancy, non-angiogenic/dormant tumors can be defined as reported in Table 1, whereas angiogenic/non-dormant tumors can be defined as shown in Table 2 [14, 20].

Metronomic Chemotherapy as an Inducer of Angiogenic Tumor Dormancy: A Promising Research Field

Metronomic chemotherapy could be defined as a frequent, regular administration of drug doses designed to maintain a low, but active, range of concentrations of chemotherapeutic drugs during prolonged periods of time without inducing excessive toxicities [43]. Various mechanisms of action of metronomic chemotherapy have been suggested for different chemotherapeutic drugs and for the same drugs but at different plasma concentrations (e.g. cyclophosphamide) [43]. This is consistent with the numerous evidences that this type of therapy is a complex approach involving both tumor cells and their microenvironment, including microvessels and cells of immune system [44].

Numerous findings support the hypothesis that metronomic chemotherapy caused antitumor effects by inhibiting tumor angiogenesis [45] because of a preferential antiendothelial activity [46]. But this is not the sole mechanism for it causing antitumor effects. There is a growing scientific literature that indicates low doses of certain chemotherapeutic drugs—especially cyclophosphamide—could cause stimulation of cytotoxic T cells by targeting T regulatory cells [47]. Metronomic chemotherapy may also have significant direct antitumor cell effects [48], also through an activity on the putative cancer stem cell (CSC) or tumor-initiating cell (TIC) subpopulation [49, 50].

Metronomic Chemotherapy and the Anti/pro-Angiogenic Growth Factor Equilibrium

As described in the previous section of this chapter, the unbalanced expression of endogenous inhibitors (e.g., TSP-1) of angiogenesis and pro-angiogenic factors (e.g. VEGF or bFGF) toward the first ones is an important characteristic of the maintenance of a dormant tumor angiogenesis [25]. Metronomic chemotherapy may be a therapeutic approach that can induce or re-induce the tumor dormancy through a marked modulation of anti- and pro-angiogenic factors (Fig. 1) both in adjuvant setting or in the treatment of metastatic disease.

Bocci and colleagues in 2003 [51] reported, for the first time, that the metronomic chemotherapy (e.g., paclitaxel, epothilones and cyclophosphamide) could induce expression of TSP-1 *in vitro* and *in vivo*. In particular, the authors demonstrated that the *in vivo* antiangiogenic and antitumor effects of daily oral metronomic cyclophosphamide were lost in TSP-1-*null* C57BL/6 mice affected by LLC, whereas, in contrast, these effects were maintained in TSP-1 *wild type* mice. More importantly, higher increases in circulating TSP-1 were detected in the plasma of responder human prostate (PC3) tumor xenograft-bearing mice treated with metronomic low-dose cyclophosphamide [51]. These findings were later confirmed using metronomic cyclophosphamide by Hamano et al. in *in vivo* models of murine cancers such as

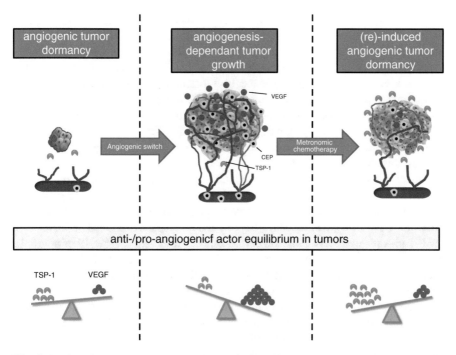

Fig. 1 Angiogenic tumor dormancy, angiogenesis-dependant tumor growth, and metronomic chemotherapy-induced angiogenic tumor dormancy. Metronomic chemotherapy modulates the equilibrium of anti- and pro-angiogenic factors in tumor microenvironment, upregulating thrombospondin-1 (TSP-1) and decreasing the vascular endothelial growth factor (VEGF). Moreover, the low-dose chemotherapy blocks the recruitment of circulating endothelial progenitors (CEPs) in the tumor mass

LLC and B16F10 melanoma [52] and by the group of Norrby in rats bearing a malignant prostate tumor (Dunning AT-1) [53], as well as by Vives and colleagues in mice with a human xenograft of ovarian cancer cell lines [54]. Moreover, also other metronomically-administered drugs were able to increase both the gene expression and the protein secretion of TSP-1 in preclinical *in vitro* and *in vivo* model. Metronomic gemcitabine was successfully used in human pancreatic adenocarcinomas xenografts, causing the reduction of tumor growth and the significant increase of TSP-1 [55, 54], whereas low dose capecitabine determined an antiangiogenic effect on human colorectal cancer COL-1 xenografts inducing TSP-1 expression in tumor tissues [56] and decreased microvessel density (MVD) in colon cancer elevating TSP-1 expression [57]. Metronomic S-1 (a 5-FU-based drug) and metronomic S-1 with vandetanib (a dual tyrosine kinase inhibitor of VEGFR-2 and EGFR) decreased MVDs and increased apoptosis in hepatocellular carcinoma tissues, upregulating the expression of TSP-1 [58]. Other examples of this phenomenon were the metronomic ceramide analogs (eg., C2 and AL6) that inhibited angiogenesis and tumor growth in pancreatic cancer through up-regulation of TSP-1 and caveolin-1 [59], whereas long term, low concentrations of SN-38 (the active metabolite of irinotecan) increased both TSP-1 gene expression and secretion by HT-29 colorectal cancer cells [60]. Finally, tubulin inhibitors such as paclitaxel and docetaxel have shown strong anti-angiogenic characteristics at low concentrations [61, 62]. In particular, low doses of paclitaxel and of its different pharmaceutical formulations (e.g. nanoparticles) determined antiangiogenic effects through the marked increase of TSP-1 levels in tumor vascular endothelial cells [63] and in different tumor types such as ovarian carcinoma [64], colon cancer [65], breast cancer [66]. Furthermore, docetaxel increased the expression of TSP-1 in a gastric cancer model [67], blocking the angiogenic process and the tumor growth.

Interestingly, this significant upregulation of TSP-1 during metronomic chemotherapy was not only limited to preclinical findings but it was also found in patients enrolled in various phase II, metronomic chemotherapy clinical trials, involving different types of cancer. Indeed, Allegrini and colleagues described an increase of TSP-1 plasma levels in metastatic colorectal cancer patients at day 49 of treatment with a continuous low dose infusion of irinotecan (1.4 and 2.8 mg/m^2/day) [68]. This finding was later confirmed in metastatic gastrointestinal cancer patients treated with a combination of metronomic cyclophosphamide (50 mg/day), UFT (100 mg/day) and celecoxib (200 mg/twice a day). Patients with a stable disease, during the metronomic schedule, had higher values of TSP-1 Area Under Curves (AUCs) if compared with patients with a progressive disease [69]. Recently, a similar result was obtained in metastatic castration-resistant prostate cancer patients treated with metronomic vinorelbine (30 mg/day p.o. thrice a week) plus 1 mg/day dexamethasone. Indeed, responder patients maintained higher plasma TSP-1 AUCs if compared to the non-responder ones [70]. Long-term oral administration of daily low-dose mercaptopurine and weekly low-dose methotrexate are used as maintenance chemotherapy in the treatment of acute lymphoblastic leukemia in children. Also this metronomic-like treatment have been described to determine a significant increase in TSP-1 plasma levels [71].

Besides the increased levels of the endogenous inhibitor of angiogenesis TSP-1, metronomic chemotherapy determine, in parallel, a well-described decrease of pro-angiogenic factor levels, such as VEGF, both in preclinical studies and in clinical trials. As such, the investigation of the antiangiogenic effects of the metronomic chemotherapy has focused on the modulation of the balance between angiogenic stimuli and natural inhibitors of angiogenesis. Indeed, another way that metronomic chemotherapy can conceivably cause an antiangiogenic effect, at least with certain drugs such as topotecan, a topoisomerase 1 inhibitor, or the anthracycline adriamycin is by suppression of the expression of HIF-1α—as originally reported by the group of Melillo and colleagues [72, 73]. HIF-1α is a known driver of VEGF-angiogenesis because it stimulates the VEGF production and secretion by hypoxic tumor cells [74]. Therefore, the pro-angiogenic VEGF levels were reduced *in vitro* in ovarian HeyA8 and SKOV3ip1 cancer cells by low concentrations of topotecan, independently of proteasome degradation and topoisomerase I inhibition [75]. Moreover, another camptothecin such as irinotecan have shown to reduce the expression of VEGF and HIF-1α in malignant glioma xenografts [76]. It has been also demonstrated that metronomic etoposide impaired the angiogenic equilibrium in tumors by inhibiting VEGF-A and FGF-2 secretion from tumor cells and by increasing endostatin plasma levels [77]. In another preclinical research performed in pancreatic cancer xenografts, metronomic gemcitabine decreased tumor levels of various proangiogenic molecules such as EGF, IL-1α, IL-8, ICAM-1, and VCAM-1 [78]. Moreover, Aktas and colleagues [79] tested lower doses of chemotherapeutic drugs such as 5-florouracil (5-FU), irinotecan, oxaliplatin, paclitaxel and docetaxel in different tumor cell lines, showing that these drugs decreased VEGF secretion from tumor cells without causing substantial cell killing. Both the expression and secretion of VEGF significantly decreased in BGC-823 gastric cancer cells treated with metronomic docetaxel [67], whereas the long term (144 h), continuous treatment with SN-38 of colon cancer cells (HT-29 and SW620) determined a significant decrease of secreted VEGF in cell media [60]. The 5-FU prodrug capecitabine metronomically administered decreased VEGF levels in *in vivo* colon cancer [57], and in gastric cancer [80] models. Furthermore, metronomic GMX1777, a chemotherapeutic drug affecting cellular energy metabolism, in a mouse model of neuroblastoma decreased stromal VEGF-A and PDGF-B mRNA in response to treatment [81]. These effects were also achieved combining different metronomic chemotherapy schedules. Mainetti and colleagues investigated the therapeutic efficacy of a combined treatment including metronomic cyclophosphamide and doxorubicin in two mouse mammary adenocarcinoma models. Interestingly, the combination was more effective than each monotherapy to decrease the VEGF serum concentration and increase tumor apoptosis [82].

Numerous phase I-II clinical studies in different types of cancer, using various chemotherapeutic drugs, have clearly suggested that plasma or serum VEGF is decreased during or after metronomic chemotherapy schedules, also combined with other drugs. In metastatic castration-resistant prostate cancer patients treated with metronomic cyclophosphamide (50 mg/day), celecoxib, and dexamethasone, the VEGF levels markedly increased in non responder subjects and remained significantly higher than in responders for more than 3 months [83]. In contrast, VEGF concentrations in responder patients constantly decreased to values corresponding to the half of the baseline [83]. Moreover, another phase II clinical trial performed in the same type of prostate cancer patients but treated with a combination of metronomic vinorelbine (30 mg/day p.o. thrice a week) plus dexamethasone, showed a plasma VEGF $AUC_{0-24day}$ significantly increased in non-responders if compared to the subjects with a PSA decrease [70]. Interestingly, germline *VEGF-A* polymorphisms predicted progression-free survival among advanced castration-resistant prostate cancer patients treated with metronomic cyclophosphamide [84]. In particular, patients harboring the *VEGF*-634CC genotype had a median progression-free survival (PFS) of 2.2 months whereas patients with the genotype -634CG/GG had a median PFS of 6.25 months ($P = 0.0042$) [84]. The decrease of plasma VEGF levels during metronomic chemotherapy have been also well described in metastatic breast cancer patients. Calleri and colleagues found out that patients affected by breast cancer with lower VEGF levels after 2 months of metronomic cyclophosphamide (50 mg/day) treatment had higher PFS, whereas at the time of progression there was a significant increase of VEGF [85]. A similar drop of serum VEGF was found in 171 metastatic breast cancer patients treated with metronomic cyclophosphamide (50 mg/day) combined with methotrexate or thalidomide after 2 months of therapy [86], whereas EL-Arab and co-workers treated the same type of patients with the combination of capecitabine (500 mg twice daily) together with oral cyclophosphamide (50 mg once daily), causing a significant decline of the median serum VEGF level after 2 and 6 months of therapy among subjects with a complete or partial response and a stable disease [87]. Interestingly, also in primary breast cancer, there was a significant suppression of VEGF-A expression in the letrozole/metronomic cyclophosphamide-treated group (50 mg/day) of patients if compared to the letrozole-treated group [88] with a lower VEGF expression at post-treatment residual histology. These data were later confirmed by Bazzola et al. who found that VEGF expression declined in tumor tissues in response to treatment with metronomic cyclophosphamide and letrozole [89]. Recently, the metronomic therapy including etoposide and cyclophosphamide determined the significant decrease of serum VEGF levels in relapsed or refractory non-Hodgkin's lymphoma patients with overall response and disease control during different cycles of therapy [90].

Metronomic Chemotherapy and the Circulating Endothelial Progenitors

Although the role of BMDC in the early stages of tumor progression is still debated, it is well accepted that the induction of angiogenesis is a key step in the progression of microtumors. Therefore, this tumors have to activate ad recruit distant and normal cells such as CEPs that will facilitate the shift toward the generation of new blood vessels [3]. The development of therapeutic approaches that are able to block and inhibit the mobilization and viability of CEPs and other pro-angiogenic BMDCs will maintain or prolong the tumor dormancy due to the angiogenesis stoppage. In this perspective, the metronomic chemotherapy could be a perfect tool to achieve this aim (Fig. 1). Indeed, it has been described that low dose chemotherapy is able to suppress the BMDC proangiogenic cells such as CEPs [44]. In 2003, there was the first evidence of this effect in mice affected by lymphoma that underwent cycles of oral low-dose cyclophosphamide therapy [91]. The metronomic schedule markedly suppressed the number of CEPs during the therapy whereas, at the end of the drug administration, the number of endothelial progenitors increased again and tumors started to grow [91]. Furthermore, 2 years later the Kerbel's team showed a clear correlation between the maximal suppression of CEP levels and the maximum antiangiogenic activity in mice treated with different drugs metronomically administered such as cyclophosphamide, vinblastine, cisplatin, or vinorelbine [92, 93]. For this reason, it has also been suggested that CEP suppression could be one of the main mechanisms of action of metronomic chemotherapy [94] and that this decline in blood of CEP levels could be used as pharmacodynamic biomarker of therapeutic efficacy [95]. Also oral metronomic topotecan in combination with pazopanib determined a significant reduction in viable CEPs as well as circulating endothelial cells (CECs), reducing the tumor MVD in several preclinical models of pediatric solid tumors [96]. The CEP percentage was found to be decreased in the peripheral blood of gastric tumor-bearing mice after the treatment with metronomic 5-FU or capecitabine [80]. Interestingly, Daenen et al. found that daily oral low-dose metronomic cyclophosphamide was capable of preventing the CEP spike and tumor colonization induced by a vascular disrupting agent if administered simultaneously [97].

Clinically, after the administration of trofosfamide-based conventional schedules of chemotherapy the numbers of circulating CEPs increased, whereas, in sharp contrast, under low-dose metronomic trofosfamide, the numbers of circulating CEPs declined significantly in blood of tumor patients [98]. Calleri and colleagues showed that in a group of 15 long-term responders to metronomic chemotherapy, there were significant trends toward lower levels of CEPs and CECs [85]. In a population of gastrointestinal cancer patients, the levels of progenitor or stem cell mRNA (i.e. CD133), during the metronomic combined treatment of UFT and cyclophosphamide, were consistently lower in those with stable disease whereas a substantial increase of CD133 gene expression was found in the progressive disease [69].

Conclusions

Angiogenic tumor dormancy occurs as a result of a dynamic equilibrium state in which antiangiogenic and pro-angiogenic stimuli are balanced and angiogenesis process is blocked. It can take place at the primary site of cancer, but also in metastatic lesions. Thus, a therapeutic approach that can achieve an induction or a "re-induction" of the angiogenic tumor dormancy in primary and/or metastatic tumors is highly welcomed in the clinical oncology field. In this perspective, metronomic chemotherapy, by upregulating the endogenous inhibitor TSP-1 and, parallely, decreasing pro-angiogenic factors or blocking CEPs, may be able to play a main role in the modulation of the angiogenic tumor dormancy. Further studies are needed to better investigate this particular aspect of this promising therapeutic tool.

Acknowledgements G.B.'s research is currently supported by grants from the Italian Association of Cancer Research (AIRC, IG 17672) and the Istituto Toscano Tumori (ITT).

References

1. Goss PE, Chambers AF (2010) Does tumour dormancy offer a therapeutic target? Nat Rev Cancer 10(12):871–877. doi:10.1038/nrc2933
2. Udagawa T (2008) Tumor dormancy of primary and secondary cancers. APMIS 116(7–8):615–628. doi:10.1111/j.1600-0463.2008.01077.x
3. Shaked Y, McAllister S, Fainaru O, Almog N (2014) Tumor dormancy and the angiogenic switch: possible implications of bone marrow-derived cells. Curr Pharm Des 20(30):4920–4933
4. Osisami M, Keller ET (2013) Mechanisms of metastatic tumor dormancy. J Clin Med 2(3):136–150. doi:10.3390/jcm2030136

5. Uhr JW, Pantel K (2011) Controversies in clinical cancer dormancy. Proc Natl Acad Sci U S A 108(30):12396–12400. doi:10.1073/pnas.1106613108
6. Aguirre-Ghiso JA (2007) Models, mechanisms and clinical evidence for cancer dormancy. Nat Rev Cancer 7(11):834–846. doi:10.1038/nrc2256
7. Favaro E, Amadori A, Indraccolo S (2008) Cellular interactions in the vascular niche: implications in the regulation of tumor dormancy. APMIS 116(7–8):648–659. doi:10.1111/j.1600-0463.2008.01025.x
8. Almog N (2010) Molecular mechanisms underlying tumor dormancy. Cancer Lett 294(2):139–146. doi:10.1016/j.canlet.2010.03.004
9. Fidler IJ (2003) The pathogenesis of cancer metastasis: the 'seed and soil' hypothesis revisited. Nat Rev Cancer 3(6):453–458. doi:10.1038/nrc1098
10. Sosa MS, Bragado P, Aguirre-Ghiso JA (2014) Mechanisms of disseminated cancer cell dormancy: an awakening field. Nat Rev Cancer 14(9):611–622. doi:10.1038/nrc3793
11. Koebel CM, Vermi W, Swann JB, Zerafa N, Rodig SJ, Old LJ, Smyth MJ, Schreiber RD (2007) Adaptive immunity maintains occult cancer in an equilibrium state. Nature 450(7171):903–907. doi:10.1038/nature06309
12. Moserle L, Amadori A, Indraccolo S (2009) The angiogenic switch: implications in the regulation of tumor dormancy. Curr Mol Med 9(8):935–941
13. Barkan D, Kleinman H, Simmons JL, Asmussen H, Kamaraju AK, Hoenorhoff MJ, Liu ZY, Costes SV, Cho EH, Lockett S, Khanna C, Chambers AF, Green JE (2008) Inhibition of metastatic outgrowth from single dormant tumor cells by targeting the cytoskeleton. Cancer Res 68(15):6241–6250. doi:10.1158/0008-5472.can-07-6849
14. Naumov GN, Folkman J, Straume O (2009) Tumor dormancy due to failure of angiogenesis: role of the microenvironment. Clin Exp Metastasis 26(1):51–60. doi:10.1007/s10585-008-9176-0
15. Naumov GN, Folkman J, Straume O, Akslen LA (2008) Tumor-vascular interactions and tumor dormancy. APMIS 116(7–8):569–585. doi:10.1111/j.1600-0463.2008.01213.x
16. Chambers AF (2009) Influence of diet on metastasis and tumor dormancy. Clin Exp Metastasis 26(1):61–66. doi:10.1007/s10585-008-9164-4
17. Siveen KS, Prabhu K, Krishnankutty R, Kuttikrishnan S, Tsakou M, Alali FQ, Dermime S, Mohammad RM, Uddin S (2017) Vascular endothelial growth factor (VEGF) signaling in tumour vascularization: potential and challenges. Curr Vasc Pharmacol. doi:10.2174/1570161115666170105124038
18. Ribatti D, Vacca A, Dammacco F (1999) The role of the vascular phase in solid tumor growth: a historical review. Neoplasia 1(4):293–302
19. Jayson GC, Kerbel R, Ellis LM, Harris AL (2016) Antiangiogenic therapy in oncology: current status and future directions. Lancet 388(10043):518–529. doi:10.1016/s0140-6736(15)01088-0
20. Naumov GN, Akslen LA, Folkman J (2006) Role of angiogenesis in human tumor dormancy: animal models of the angiogenic switch. Cell Cycle 5(16):1779–1787. doi:10.4161/cc.5.16.3018
21. Folkman J (1971) Tumor angiogenesis: therapeutic implications. N Engl J Med 285(21):1182–1186. doi:10.1056/nejm197111182852108
22. Natale G, Bocci G, Lenzi P (2017) Looking for the word "angiogenesis" in the history of health sciences: from ancient times to the first decades of the twentieth century. World J Surg 41(6):1625–1634. doi: 10.1007/s00268-016-3680-1
23. Katoh M (2016) Therapeutics targeting FGF signaling network in human diseases. Trends Pharmacol Sci 37(12):1081–1096. doi:10.1016/j.tips.2016.10.003
24. Dewerchin M, Carmeliet P (2014) Placental growth factor in cancer. Expert Opin Ther Targets 18(11):1339–1354. doi:10.1517/14728222.2014.948420
25. Kang SY, Watnick RS (2008) Regulation of tumor dormancy as a function of tumor-mediated paracrine regulation of stromal tsp-1 and VEGF expression. APMIS 116(7–8):638–647. doi:10.1111/j.1600-0463.2008.01138.x
26. Gacche RN, Meshram RJ (2013) Targeting tumor micro-environment for design and development of novel anti-angiogenic agents arresting tumor growth. Prog Biophys Mol Biol 113(2):333–354. doi:10.1016/j.pbiomolbio.2013.10.001

27. Rak J, Mitsuhashi Y, Bayko L, Filmus J, Shirasawa S, Sasazuki T, Kerbel RS (1995) Mutant ras oncogenes upregulate VEGF/VPF expression: implications for induction and inhibition of tumor angiogenesis. Cancer Res 55(20):4575–4580
28. Achilles EG, Fernandez A, Allred EN, Kisker O, Udagawa T, Beecken WD, Flynn E, Folkman J (2001) Heterogeneity of angiogenic activity in a human liposarcoma: a proposed mechanism for "no take" of human tumors in mice. J Natl Cancer Inst 93(14):1075–1081
29. Pugh CW, Ratcliffe PJ (2003) Regulation of angiogenesis by hypoxia: role of the HIF system. Nat Med 9(6):677–684. doi:10.1038/nm0603-677
30. Naumov GN, Bender E, Zurakowski D, Kang SY, Sampson D, Flynn E, Watnick RS, Straume O, Akslen LA, Folkman J, Almog N (2006) A model of human tumor dormancy: an angiogenic switch from the nonangiogenic phenotype. J Natl Cancer Inst 98(5):316–325. doi:10.1093/jnci/djj068
31. Almog N, Ma L, Raychowdhury R, Schwager C, Erber R, Short S, Hlatky L, Vajkoczy P, Huber PE, Folkman J, Abdollahi A (2009) Transcriptional switch of dormant tumors to fast-growing angiogenic phenotype. Cancer Res 69(3):836–844. doi:10.1158/0008-5472.can-08-2590
32. Panigrahy D, Edin ML, Lee CR, Huang S, Bielenberg DR, Butterfield CE, Barnes CM, Mammoto A, Mammoto T, Luria A, Benny O, Chaponis DM, Dudley AC, Greene ER, Vergilio JA, Pietramaggiori G, Scherer-Pietramaggiori SS, Short SM, Seth M, Lih FB, Tomer KB, Yang J, Schwendener RA, Hammock BD, Falck JR, Manthati VL, Ingber DE, Kaipainen A, D'Amore PA, Kieran MW, Zeldin DC (2012) Epoxyeicosanoids stimulate multiorgan metastasis and tumor dormancy escape in mice. J Clin Invest 122(1):178–191. doi:10.1172/jci58128
33. Indraccolo S (2013) Insights into the regulation of tumor dormancy by angiogenesis in experimental tumors. Adv Exp Med Biol 734:37–52. doi:10.1007/978-1-4614-1445-2
34. Indraccolo S, Minuzzo S, Masiero M, Pusceddu I, Persano L, Moserle L, Reboldi A, Favaro E, Mecarozzi M, Di Mario G, Screpanti I, Ponzoni M, Doglioni C, Amadori A (2009) Cross-talk between tumor and endothelial cells involving the Notch3-Dll4 interaction marks escape from tumor dormancy. Cancer Res 69(4):1314–1323. doi:10.1158/0008-5472.can-08-2791
35. Rak J, Milsom C, Yu J (2008) Vascular determinants of cancer stem cell dormancy—do age and coagulation system play a role? APMIS 116(7–8):660–676. doi:10.1111/j.1600-0463.2008.01058.x
36. Indraccolo S, Favaro E, Amadori A (2006) Dormant tumors awaken by a short-term angiogenic burst: the spike hypothesis. Cell Cycle 5(16):1751–1755. doi:10.4161/cc.5.16.2985
37. Mowers EE, Sharifi MN, Macleod KF (2017) Autophagy in cancer metastasis. Oncogene 36(12):1619–1630. doi: 10.1038/onc.2016.333
38. Grange C, Tapparo M, Collino F, Vitillo L, Damasco C, Deregibus MC, Tetta C, Bussolati B, Camussi G (2011) Microvesicles released from human renal cancer stem cells stimulate angiogenesis and formation of lung premetastatic niche. Cancer Res 71(15):5346–5356. doi:10.1158/0008-5472.can-11-0241
39. Elkabets M, Gifford AM, Scheel C, Nilsson B, Reinhardt F, Bray MA, Carpenter AE, Jirstrom K, Magnusson K, Ebert BL, Ponten F, Weinberg RA, McAllister SS (2011) Human tumors instigate granulin-expressing hematopoietic cells that promote malignancy by activating stromal fibroblasts in mice. J Clin Invest 121(2):784–799. doi:10.1172/jci43757
40. Png KJ, Halberg N, Yoshida M, Tavazoie SF (2011) A microRNA regulon that mediates endothelial recruitment and metastasis by cancer cells. Nature 481(7380):190–194. doi:10.1038/nature10661
41. Straume O, Shimamura T, Lampa MJ, Carretero J, Oyan AM, Jia D, Borgman CL, Soucheray M, Downing SR, Short SM, Kang SY, Wang S, Chen L, Collett K, Bachmann I, Wong KK, Shapiro GI, Kalland KH, Folkman J, Watnick RS, Akslen LA, Naumov GN (2012) Suppression of heat shock protein 27 induces long-term dormancy in human breast cancer. Proc Natl Acad Sci U S A 109(22):8699–8704. doi:10.1073/pnas.1017909109
42. Almog N, Ma L, Schwager C, Brinkmann BG, Beheshti A, Vajkoczy P, Folkman J, Hlatky L, Abdollahi A (2012) Consensus micro RNAs governing the switch of dormant tumors to the fast-growing angiogenic phenotype. PLoS One 7(8):e44001. doi:10.1371/journal.pone.0044001

43. Bocci G, Kerbel RS (2016) Pharmacokinetics of metronomic chemotherapy: a neglected but crucial aspect. Nat Rev Clin Oncol 13(11):659–673. doi:10.1038/nrclinonc.2016.64
44. Pasquier E, Kavallaris M, Andre N (2010) Metronomic chemotherapy: new rationale for new directions. Nat Rev Clin Oncol 7(8):455–465. doi:10.1038/nrclinonc.2010.82
45. Penel N, Adenis A, Bocci G (2012) Cyclophosphamide-based metronomic chemotherapy: after 10 years of experience, where do we stand and where are we going? Crit Rev Oncol Hematol 82(1):40–50. doi:10.1016/j.critrevonc.2011.04.009
46. Bocci G, Nicolaou KC, Kerbel RS (2002) Protracted low-dose effects on human endothelial cell proliferation and survival in vitro reveal a selective antiangiogenic window for various chemotherapeutic drugs. Cancer Res 62(23):6938–6943
47. Ghiringhelli F, Menard C, Puig PE, Ladoire S, Roux S, Martin F, Solary E, Le Cesne A, Zitvogel L, Chauffert B (2007) Metronomic cyclophosphamide regimen selectively depletes CD4+CD25+ regulatory T cells and restores T and NK effector functions in end stage cancer patients. Cancer Immunol Immunother 56(5):641–648. doi:10.1007/s00262-006-0225-8
48. Fioravanti A, Canu B, Ali G, Orlandi P, Allegrini G, Di Desidero T, Emmenegger U, Fontanini G, Danesi R, Del Tacca M, Falcone A, Bocci G (2009) Metronomic 5-fluorouracil, oxali-platin and irinotecan in colorectal cancer. Eur J Pharmacol 619(1–3):8–14. doi:10.1016/j.ejphar.2009.08.020
49. Folkins C, Shaked Y, Man S, Tang T, Lee CR, Zhu Z, Hoffman RM, Kerbel RS (2009) Glioma tumor stem-like cells promote tumor angiogenesis and vasculogenesis via vascular endothelial growth factor and stromal-derived factor 1. Cancer Res 69(18):7243–7251. doi:10.1158/0008-5472.can-09-0167
50. Chan TS, Hsu CC, Pai VC, Liao WY, Huang SS, Tan KT, Yen CJ, Hsu SC, Chen WY, Shan YS, Li CR, Lee MT, Jiang KY, Chu JM, Lien GS, Weaver VM, Tsai KK (2016) Metronomic chemotherapy prevents therapy-induced stromal activation and induction of tumor-initiating cells. J Exp Med 213(13):2967–2988. doi:10.1084/jem.20151665
51. Bocci G, Francia G, Man S, Lawler J, Kerbel RS (2003) Thrombospondin 1, a mediator of the antiangiogenic effects of low-dose metronomic chemotherapy. Proc Natl Acad Sci U S A 100(22):12917–12922. doi:10.1073/pnas.2135406100
52. Hamano Y, Sugimoto H, Soubasakos MA, Kieran M, Olsen BR, Lawler J, Sudhakar A, Kalluri R (2004) Thrombospondin-1 associated with tumor microenvironment contributes to low-dose cyclophosphamide-mediated endothelial cell apoptosis and tumor growth suppression. Cancer Res 64(5):1570–1574
53. Damber JE, Vallbo C, Albertsson P, Lennernas B, Norrby K (2006) The anti-tumour effect of low-dose continuous chemotherapy may partly be mediated by thrombospondin. Cancer Chemother Pharmacol 58(3):354–360. doi:10.1007/s00280-005-0163-8
54. Vives M, Ginesta MM, Gracova K, Graupera M, Casanovas O, Capella G, Serrano T, Laquente B, Vinals F (2013) Metronomic chemotherapy following the maximum tolerated dose is an effective anti-tumour therapy affecting angiogenesis, tumour dissemination and cancer stem cells. Int J Cancer 133(10):2464–2472. doi:10.1002/ijc.28259
55. Laquente B, Lacasa C, Ginesta MM, Casanovas O, Figueras A, Galan M, Ribas IG, Germa JR, Capella G, Vinals F (2008) Antiangiogenic effect of gemcitabine following metronomic administration in a pancreas cancer model. Mol Cancer Ther 7(3):638–647. doi:10.1158/1535-7163.mct-07-2122
56. Ooyama A, Oka T, Zhao HY, Yamamoto M, Akiyama S, Fukushima M (2008) Anti-angiogenic effect of 5-fluorouracil-based drugs against human colon cancer xenografts. Cancer Lett 267(1):26–36. doi:10.1016/j.canlet.2008.03.008
57. Shi H, Jiang J, Ji J, Shi M, Cai Q, Chen X, Yu Y, Liu B, Zhu Z, Zhang J (2014) Anti-angiogenesis participates in antitumor effects of metronomic capecitabine on colon cancer. Cancer Lett 349(2):128–135. doi:10.1016/j.canlet.2014.04.002
58. Iwamoto H, Torimura T, Nakamura T, Hashimoto O, Inoue K, Kurogi J, Niizeki T, Kuwahara R, Abe M, Koga H, Yano H, Kerbel RS, Ueno T, Sata M (2011) Metronomic S-1 chemotherapy and vandetanib: an efficacious and nontoxic treatment for hepatocellular carcinoma. Neoplasia 13(3):187–197

59. Bocci G, Fioravanti A, Orlandi P, Di Desidero T, Natale G, Fanelli G, Viacava P, Naccarato AG, Francia G, Danesi R (2012) Metronomic ceramide analogs inhibit angiogenesis in pancreatic cancer through up-regulation of caveolin-1 and thrombospondin-1 and down-regulation of cyclin D1. Neoplasia 14(9):833–845

60. Bocci G, Falcone A, Fioravanti A, Orlandi P, Di Paolo A, Fanelli G, Viacava P, Naccarato AG, Kerbel RS, Danesi R, Del Tacca M, Allegrini G (2008) Antiangiogenic and anticolorectal cancer effects of metronomic irinotecan chemotherapy alone and in combination with semaxinib. Br J Cancer 98(10):1619–1629. doi:10.1038/sj.bjc.6604352

61. Bocci G, Di Paolo A, Danesi R (2013) The pharmacological bases of the antiangiogenic activity of paclitaxel. Angiogenesis 16(3):481–492. doi:10.1007/s10456-013-9334-0

62. Pasquier E, Andre N, Braguer D (2007) Targeting microtubules to inhibit angiogenesis and disrupt tumour vasculature: implications for cancer treatment. Curr Cancer Drug Targets 7(6):566–581

63. Luan X, Guan YY, Lovell JF, Zhao M, Lu Q, Liu YR, Liu HJ, Gao YG, Dong X, Yang SC, Zheng L, Sun P, Fang C, Chen HZ (2016) Tumor priming using metronomic chemotherapy with neovasculature-targeted, nanoparticulate paclitaxel. Biomaterials 95:60–73. doi:10.1016/j.biomaterials.2016.04.008

64. Lee SJ, Ghosh SC, Han HD, Stone RL, Bottsford-Miller J, Shen DY, Auzenne EJ, Lopez-Araujo A, Lu C, Nishimura M, Pecot CV, Zand B, Thanapprapasr D, Jennings NB, Kang Y, Huang J, Hu W, Klostergaard J, Sood AK (2012) Metronomic activity of CD44-targeted hyaluronic acid-paclitaxel in ovarian carcinoma. Clin Cancer Res 18(15):4114–4121. doi:10.1158/1078-0432.ccr-11-3250

65. Zhang M, Tao W, Pan S, Sun X, Jiang H (2009) Low-dose metronomic chemotherapy of paclitaxel synergizes with cetuximab to suppress human colon cancer xenografts. Anti-Cancer Drugs 20(5):355–363. doi:10.1097/CAD.0b013e3283299f36

66. Tao WY, Liang XS, Liu Y, Wang CY, Pang D (2015) Decrease of let-7f in low-dose metronomic paclitaxel chemotherapy contributed to upregulation of thrombospondin-1 in breast cancer. Int J Biol Sci 11(1):48–58. doi:10.7150/ijbs.9969

67. Wu H, Xin Y, Zhao J, Sun D, Li W, Hu Y, Wang S (2011) Metronomic docetaxel chemotherapy inhibits angiogenesis and tumor growth in a gastric cancer model. Cancer Chemother Pharmacol 68(4):879–887. doi:10.1007/s00280-011-1563-6

68. Allegrini G, Falcone A, Fioravanti A, Barletta MT, Orlandi P, Loupakis F, Cerri E, Masi G, Di Paolo A, Kerbel RS, Danesi R, Del Tacca M, Bocci G (2008) A pharmacokinetic and pharmacodynamic study on metronomic irinotecan in metastatic colorectal cancer patients. Br J Cancer 98(8):1312–1319. doi:10.1038/sj.bjc.6604311

69. Allegrini G, Di Desidero T, Barletta MT, Fioravanti A, Orlandi P, Canu B, Chericoni S, Loupakis F, Di Paolo A, Masi G, Fontana A, Lucchesi S, Arrighi G, Giusiani M, Ciarlo A, Brandi G, Danesi R, Kerbel RS, Falcone A, Bocci G (2012) Clinical, pharmacokinetic and pharmacodynamic evaluations of metronomic UFT and cyclophosphamide plus celecoxib in patients with advanced refractory gastrointestinal cancers. Angiogenesis 15(2):275–286. doi:10.1007/s10456-012-9260-6

70. Di Desidero T, Derosa L, Galli L, Orlandi P, Fontana A, Fioravanti A, Marconcini R, Giorgi M, Campi B, Saba A, Lucchesi S, Felipetto R, Danesi R, Francia G, Allegrini G, Falcone A, Bocci G (2016) Clinical, pharmacodynamic and pharmacokinetic results of a prospective phase II study on oral metronomic vinorelbine and dexamethasone in castration-resistant prostate cancer patients. Investig New Drugs 34(6):760–770. doi:10.1007/s10637-016-0385-0

71. Andre N, Cointe S, Barlogis V, Arnaud L, Lacroix R, Pasquier E, Dignat-George F, Michel G, Sabatier F (2015) Maintenance chemotherapy in children with ALL exerts metronomic-like thrombospondin-1 associated anti-endothelial effect. Oncotarget 6(26):23008–23014. doi:10.18632/oncotarget.3984

72. Calvani M, Rapisarda A, Uranchimeg B, Shoemaker RH, Melillo G (2006) Hypoxic induction of an HIF-1alpha-dependent bFGF autocrine loop drives angiogenesis in human endothelial cells. Blood 107(7):2705–2712. doi:10.1182/blood-2005-09-3541

73. Rapisarda A, Zalek J, Hollingshead M, Braunschweig T, Uranchimeg B, Bonomi CA, Borgel SD, Carter JP, Hewitt SM, Shoemaker RH, Melillo G (2004) Schedule-dependent inhibition of hypoxia-inducible factor-1alpha protein accumulation, angiogenesis, and tumor growth by topotecan in U251-HRE glioblastoma xenografts. Cancer Res 64(19):6845–6848. doi:10.1158/0008-5472.can-04-2116

74. Masoud GN, Li W (2015) HIF-1alpha pathway: role, regulation and intervention for cancer therapy. Acta Pharm Sin B 5(5):378–389. doi:10.1016/j.apsb.2015.05.007

75. Merritt WM, Danes CG, Shahzad MM, Lin YG, Kamat AA, Han LY, Spannuth WA, Nick AM, Mangala LS, Stone RL, Kim HS, Gershenson DM, Jaffe RB, Coleman RL, Chandra J, Sood AK (2009) Anti-angiogenic properties of metronomic topotecan in ovarian carcinoma. Cancer Biol Ther 8(16):1596–1603

76. Takano S, Kamiyama H, Mashiko R, Osuka S, Ishikawa E, Matsumura A (2010) Metronomic treatment of malignant glioma xenografts with irinotecan (CPT-11) inhibits angiogenesis and tumor growth. J Neuro-Oncol 99(2):177–185. doi:10.1007/s11060-010-0118-8

77. Panigrahy D, Kaipainen A, Butterfield CE, Chaponis DM, Laforme AM, Folkman J, Kieran MW (2010) Inhibition of tumor angiogenesis by oral etoposide. Exp Ther Med 1(5):739–746. doi:10.3892/etm.2010.127

78. Cham KK, Baker JH, Takhar KS, Flexman JA, Wong MQ, Owen DA, Yung A, Kozlowski P, Reinsberg SA, Chu EM, Chang CW, Buczkowski AK, Chung SW, Scudamore CH, Minchinton AI, Yapp DT, Ng SS (2010) Metronomic gemcitabine suppresses tumour growth, improves perfusion, and reduces hypoxia in human pancreatic ductal adenocarcinoma. Br J Cancer 103(1):52–60. doi:10.1038/sj.bjc.6605727

79. Aktas SH, Akbulut H, Akgun N, Icli F (2012) Low dose chemotherapeutic drugs without overt cytotoxic effects decrease the secretion of VEGF by cultured human tumor cells: a tentative relationship between drug type and tumor cell type response. Cancer Biomark 12(3):135–140. doi:10.3233/cbm-130301

80. Yuan F, Shi H, Ji J, Cai Q, Chen X, Yu Y, Liu B, Zhu Z, Zhang J (2015) Capecitabine metronomic chemotherapy inhibits the proliferation of gastric cancer cells through anti-angiogenesis. Oncol Rep 33(4):1753–1762. doi:10.3892/or.2015.3765

81. Fuchs D, Rodriguez A, Eriksson S, Christofferson R, Sundberg C, Azarbayjani F (2010) Metronomic administration of the drug GMX1777, a cellular NAD synthesis inhibitor, results in neuroblastoma regression and vessel maturation without inducing drug resistance. Int J Cancer 126(12):2773–2789. doi:10.1002/ijc.25206

82. Mainetti LE, Rico MJ, Fernandez-Zenobi MV, Perroud HA, Roggero EA, Rozados VR, Scharovsky OG (2013) Therapeutic efficacy of metronomic chemotherapy with cyclophosphamide and doxorubicin on murine mammary adenocarcinomas. Ann Oncol 24(9):2310–2316. doi:10.1093/annonc/mdt164

83. Fontana A, Galli L, Fioravanti A, Orlandi P, Galli C, Landi L, Bursi S, Allegrini G, Fontana E, Di Marsico R, Antonuzzo A, D'Arcangelo M, Danesi R, Del Tacca M, Falcone A, Bocci G (2009) Clinical and pharmacodynamic evaluation of metronomic cyclophosphamide, celecoxib, and dexamethasone in advanced hormone-refractory prostate cancer. Clin Cancer Res 15(15):4954–4962. doi:10.1158/1078-0432.ccr-08-3317

84. Orlandi P, Fontana A, Fioravanti A, Di Desidero T, Galli L, Derosa L, Canu B, Marconcini R, Biasco E, Solini A, Francia G, Danesi R, Falcone A, Bocci G (2013) VEGF-A polymorphisms predict progression-free survival among advanced castration-resistant prostate cancer patients treated with metronomic cyclophosphamide. Br J Cancer 109(4):957–964. doi:10.1038/bjc.2013.398

85. Calleri A, Bono A, Bagnardi V, Quarna J, Mancuso P, Rabascio C, Dellapasqua S, Campagnoli E, Shaked Y, Goldhirsch A, Colleoni M, Bertolini F (2009) Predictive potential of angiogenic growth factors and circulating endothelial cells in breast cancer patients receiving metronomic chemotherapy plus bevacizumab. Clin Cancer Res 15(24):7652–7657. doi:10.1158/1078-0432.ccr-09-1493

86. Colleoni M, Orlando L, Sanna G, Rocca A, Maisonneuve P, Peruzzotti G, Ghisini R, Sandri MT, Zorzino L, Nole F, Viale G, Goldhirsch A (2006) Metronomic low-dose oral cyclophosphamide and methotrexate plus or minus thalidomide in metastatic breast cancer: antitumor activity and biological effects. Ann Oncol 17(2):232–238. doi:10.1093/annonc/mdj066
87. El-Arab LR, Swellam M, El Mahdy MM (2012) Metronomic chemotherapy in metastatic breast cancer: impact on VEGF. J Egypt Natl Canc Inst 24(1):15–22. doi:10.1016/j.jnci.2011.12.002
88. Bottini A, Generali D, Brizzi MP, Fox SB, Bersiga A, Bonardi S, Allevi G, Aguggini S, Bodini G, Milani M, Dionisio R, Bernardi C, Montruccoli A, Bruzzi P, Harris AL, Dogliotti L, Berruti A (2006) Randomized phase II trial of letrozole and letrozole plus low-dose metronomic oral cyclophosphamide as primary systemic treatment in elderly breast cancer patients. J Clin Oncol 24(22):3623–3628. doi:10.1200/jco.2005.04.5773
89. Bazzola L, Foroni C, Andreis D, Zanoni V, RC M, Allevi G, Aguggini S, Strina C, Milani M, Venturini S, Ferrozzi F, Giardini R, Bertoni R, Turley H, Gatter K, Petronini PG, Fox SB, Harris AL, Martinotti M, Berruti A, Bottini A, Reynolds AR, Generali D (2015) Combination of letrozole, metronomic cyclophosphamide and sorafenib is well-tolerated and shows activity in patients with primary breast cancer. Br J Cancer 112(1):52–60. doi:10.1038/bjc.2014.563
90. Zeng J, Yang L, Huang F, Hong T, He Z, Lei J, Sun H, Lu Y, Hao X (2016) The metronomic therapy with prednisone, etoposide, and cyclophosphamide reduces the serum levels of VEGF and circulating endothelial cells and improves response rates and progression-free survival in patients with relapsed or refractory non-Hodgkin's lymphoma. Cancer Chemother Pharmacol 78(4):801–808. doi:10.1007/s00280-016-3136-1
91. Bertolini F, Paul S, Mancuso P, Monestiroli S, Gobbi A, Shaked Y, Kerbel RS (2003) Maximum tolerable dose and low-dose metronomic chemotherapy have opposite effects on the mobilization and viability of circulating endothelial progenitor cells. Cancer Res 63(15):4342–4346
92. Shaked Y, Bertolini F, Man S, Rogers MS, Cervi D, Foutz T, Rawn K, Voskas D, Dumont DJ, Ben-David Y, Lawler J, Henkin J, Huber J, Hicklin DJ, D'Amato RJ, Kerbel RS (2005) Genetic heterogeneity of the vasculogenic phenotype parallels angiogenesis: implications for cellular surrogate marker analysis of antiangiogenesis. Cancer Cell 7(1):101–111. doi:10.1016/j.ccr.2004.11.023
93. Shaked Y, Emmenegger U, Francia G, Chen L, Lee CR, Man S, Paraghamian A, Ben-David Y, Kerbel RS (2005) Low-dose metronomic combined with intermittent bolus-dose cyclophosphamide is an effective long-term chemotherapy treatment strategy. Cancer Res 65(16):7045–7051. doi:10.1158/0008-5472.can-05-0765
94. Shaked Y, Emmenegger U, Man S, Cervi D, Bertolini F, Ben-David Y, Kerbel RS (2005) Optimal biologic dose of metronomic chemotherapy regimens is associated with maximum antiangiogenic activity. Blood 106(9):3058–3061. doi:10.1182/blood-2005-04-1422
95. Shaked Y, Bocci G, Munoz R, Man S, Ebos JM, Hicklin DJ, Bertolini F, D'Amato R, Kerbel RS (2005) Cellular and molecular surrogate markers to monitor targeted and non-targeted antiangiogenic drug activity and determine optimal biologic dose. Curr Cancer Drug Targets 5(7):551–559
96. Kumar S, Mokhtari RB, Sheikh R, Wu B, Zhang L, Xu P, Man S, Oliveira ID, Yeger H, Kerbel RS, Baruchel S (2011) Metronomic oral topotecan with pazopanib is an active antiangiogenic regimen in mouse models of aggressive pediatric solid tumor. Clin Cancer Res 17(17):5656–5667. doi:10.1158/1078-0432.ccr-11-0078
97. Daenen LG, Shaked Y, Man S, Xu P, Voest EE, Hoffman RM, Chaplin DJ, Kerbel RS (2009) Low-dose metronomic cyclophosphamide combined with vascular disrupting therapy induces potent antitumor activity in preclinical human tumor xenograft models. Mol Cancer Ther 8(10):2872–2881. doi:10.1158/1535-7163.mct-09-0583
98. Stoelting S, Trefzer T, Kisro J, Steinke A, Wagner T, Peters SO (2008) Low-dose oral metronomic chemotherapy prevents mobilization of endothelial progenitor cells into the blood of cancer patients. In Vivo 22(6):831–836

Immuno-oncology of Dormant Tumours

Noushin Nabavi, Morgan E. Roberts, Francesco Crea,
Colin C. Collins, Yuzhuo Wang, and Jennifer L. Bishop

Abstract Cancer is a complex, often aggressive disease. As such, cancer treatment requires a diverse approach that often includes surgery, chemotherapy, radiotherapy, targeted therapy, or immunotherapy. Despite the potency of these treatments, cancer cells adapt to escape killing and survive either in their original microenvironmental niche, or as disseminated cancer cells in distant organs. Depending on tumour type and treatment modality, tumours display a variety of growth patterns, from rapid proliferation and invasion to a more controlled dormant phenotype. This dormant phenotype is characterized clinically as the asymptomatic period post therapy before relapse, and biologically by an enrichment in cancer cells that are not dividing but survive in a quiescent state, arrested in G0-G1 phase of cell cycle. Dormancy is a tumour intrinsic characteristic that corresponds to the equilibrium phase of the immune-editing hypothesis, in which tumour cells neither proliferate nor are eliminated by the immune response. In this chapter we provide an overview of anti-tumour immunity and ways in which the immune response may shape tumour dormancy.

Keywords Cancer immunoediting • Immunosurveillance • Immunotherapy • Microenvironment • Cancer-immune system interactions • Immune evasion • Tumour dormancy • Therapy induced dormancy • Immune checkpoint • Checkpoint blockade

N. Nabavi (✉) • Y. Wang
Department of Experimental Therapeutics and Department of Urologic Sciences,
BC Cancer Agency and University of British Columbia, Vancouver, BC, Canada
e-mail: nnabavi@prostatecentre.com

M.E. Roberts • J.L. Bishop
Vancouver Prostate Centre, 2660 Oak Street, Vancouver, BC, Canada, V6H 3Z6
e-mail: nnabavi@prostatecentre.com

F. Crea
School of Life, Health & Chemical Sciences, The Open University, Walton Hall, Milton
Keynes, Buckinghamshire, UK

C.C. Collins
Laboratory for Advanced Genome Analysis, Vancouver Prostate Centre, 2660 Oak St,
Vancouver, BC, Canada, V6H 3Z6

Department of Urologic Sciences, University of British Columbia, 2329 West Mall,
Vancouver, BC, Canada, V6T 1Z4

© Springer International Publishing AG 2017
Y. Wang, F. Crea (eds.), *Tumor Dormancy and Recurrence*, Cancer Drug
Discovery and Development, DOI 10.1007/978-3-319-59242-8_4

51

Anti-cancer Immunity: An Overview

The immune system is an intricate and organized system of cells and organs that functions to protect the body from pathogens. Healthy immunity is achieved when cells of both the innate and adaptive arms of the immune system are able to prevent disease while avoiding destruction of host tissue, or auto-immunity. This "tolerance" of self is essential in a properly functioning immune system, yet it also poses a significant challenge to mounting an immune response against cancer, which arises from self-tissues.

Despite sharing many characteristics of normal tissue, tumour cells do express and produce antigens that are recognized as foreign by the immune response. In the 1950s, Burnet and Thomas were the first to propose that the immune system is able to detect and prevent the growth of tumours; this was the cancer immunosurveillance hypothesis [1]. It took almost 50 years and the development of highly sophisticated transgenic mouse models, where select components of the immune response could be manipulated, to prove that both innate and adaptive immunity are essential to prevent a variety of tumour types. In the early 2000s, the cancer immunosurveillance hypothesis was refined and concept of cancer immunoediting emerged. This process includes three distinct phases; i) elimination, in which cancer cells are recognized and destroyed by immune cells, ii) equilibrium, in which cancer cells survive and may be recognized by the immune response but are not eliminated by them, and iii) escape, in which the immune response is no longer able to prevent cancer cell proliferation or metastasis [2], (also depicted in Fig. 1). In the equilibrium phase, a tumour microenvironment (TME) consisting of tumour cells, immune and non-immune stromal cells, and their secreted products, is established that plays a large role in dictating whether tumours will eventually escape the immune response.

Many components of the immune system contribute to an effective anti-cancer immune response, however CD8+ cytotoxic T cells have emerged as a major driver of tumour rejection, through the direct killing of tumour cells. Induction of an effective CD8+ T cell response is a multistep process that requires coordinated interactions between numerous cell types [3, 4]. This process begins with the expression of tumour antigens that can be taken up by antigen presenting cells (APC) such as dendritic cells (DCs) and presented in the context of major histocompatibility complex (MHC). These APCs then migrate to draining lymph nodes and present the antigen to a T cell that expresses a T cell receptor (TCR) specific for that antigen-MHC complex. Effective T cell priming and activation depends on the presentation of antigen with concomitant co-stimulatory and cytokine signals, and leads to the proliferation and clonal expansion of tumour-antigen specific effector T cells. Activated T cells then travel via the bloodstream and infiltrate vascularized tumours where they recognize and kill tumour cells.

Each of these steps is carefully controlled by multiple mechanisms of immune-regulation [1, 2, 5–9], many of which may be co-opted by tumours enabling immune escape. Escape from equilibrium depends on both tumour intrinsic mechanisms of immune evasion and mechanisms of immunological tolerance [10, 11]. For example, tumours secrete multiple factors that have pleiotropic suppressive effects on

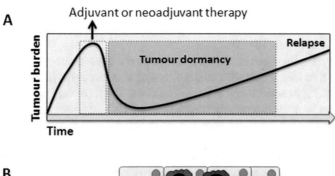

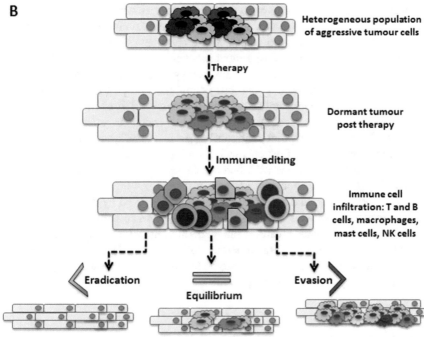

Fig. 1 (**a**) Tumour burden and volume decreases following adjuvant or neoadjuvant therapy prior to tumour recurrence, a period signified as tumour dormancy. (**b**) Cancer stem cell like interactions with immune system. The three stages of cancer immunoediting involved in growth of clinical tumours describe the intricate relationship between a tumour mass and its infiltrating immune cells. The three phases of editing consist of eradication, equilibrium, and escape. Eradication: Highly immunogenic tumour cells are eradicated by an armamentaria of immune cells. Equilibrium: Moderately immunogenic tumour cells are partially eradicated by immune cells and some remain dormant. Evasion: Poorly immunogenic tumour cells evade immunosurveillance and invade their microenvironment

immune cells in the TME. While cytokines and growth factors like IL-1β, GM-CSF, and VEGF have been implicated in driving the expansion of myeloid derived suppressor cells (MDSCs) within the TME that promote tumour growth [12], others like TGF-β [13] and IDO [14] secreted by DCs play important roles in the conversion of effector CD4+ T cells towards a T regulatory (Treg) cell phenotype. The accumulation of MDSCs and Treg cells within the TME is a poor prognostic indicator across multiple cancer types [15–18].

Tumour intrinsic mechanisms of immune escape also include the expression of surface molecules that interact directly with infiltrating immune cells, thereby preventing their activation or anti-tumour effector functions. The most well studied are Ig family molecules such as programmed death ligand-1 (PD-L1), which acts as an inhibitory signal when bound to its receptor, programmed cell death 1 (PD-1), expressed on activated T cells, natural killer (NK) cells, B cells and some myeloid subsets. Overall, immune escape occurs as a result of induction of potent immunosuppressive mechanisms, or through immune editing, in which the immune system kills immunogenic tumour clones effectively selecting for cancer cells that are non-immunogenic and fall "under the radar" of immune surveillance.

The clinical significance of the tumour immunosurveillance is highlighted by the increased incidence of cancer in patients undergoing immunosuppressive therapy [19, 20]. Furthermore, the effective use of immunotherapies targeting inhibitory receptors, so called checkpoint molecules, that limit T cell effector activity, have now re-established the capacity of the immune system to effectively eradicate tumours. The use of checkpoint inhibitors has led to dramatic and long-lasting clinical responses in a subset of patients with a variety of cancers, including metastatic melanoma and bladder cancer [21]. Indeed, anti-cytotoxic T lymphocyte associated protein 4 (CTLA-4) monoclonal antibodies (mAb) (ipilimumab), and anti-PD-1 mAb (pembrolizumab and nivolumab) have been approved by the FDA for use in metastatic melanoma, while the anti-PD-L1 mAb (atezolizumab) has been approved for use in metastatic bladder cancer, and numerous clinical trials are currently ongoing [11, 21]. This, together with numerous studies identifying positive associations between tumour immune infiltrates with better prognosis, highlight the importance of the immune system in regulating cancer progression [22, 23].

Dormant Tumour-Immune System Interactions

Tumour dormancy can exist as either a state in which rates of cell proliferation match those of cell death, or when tumour cells themselves are in a state of quiescence [10]. Dormant tumour cells are by default in a state of equilibrium with the immune response. In the context of the immune-editing hypothesis, tumour cells exiting dormancy will therefore be either eliminated by, or escape anti-tumour immunity. The length of the dormancy equilibrium period, signified with minimal residual diseased-state, depends on the patient and cancer type [24, 25]. Prostate [26], breast [27], melanoma [28], and non-hodgkin's lymphoma [29] patients show relatively longer disease free periods post therapy prior to recurrence compared to higher mortality cancers of pancreas [30], brain [31], lung [32] and esophagus [33]. Importantly, although dormant tumours are in equilibrium with immune responses and tumour cells exiting dormancy must evade or trigger immune responses, the variability in dormancy periods across cancers cannot be explained by one "immune-phenotype". Indeed, how dormant tumour cells specifically interact with immune cells at this stage remains unclear.

The value of immunity directed against cancer stem cells (CSCs) however, is an area of rapidly expanding research that may provide insight as to how dormant cells, which share many features of CSCs in terms of their microenvironmental niche and survival mechanisms [34, 35], induce or prevent immune responses. CSCs across multiple tumour types alter cell surface molecules known to inhibit both innate and adaptive anti-tumour immunity, including the anti-phagocytosis receptor CD47 [36], MHC I [37], MHC II [38], and PD-L1 [39–42]. In certain CSC types, tumour neoantigens are also expressed at lower levels compared to non-CSCs, and induce expansion of Treg cells [43]. CSCs in renal cell carcinoma have also been shown to prevent the differentiation of mature DCs [44].

Despite these immune evasion strategies, CSCs express multiple tumour associated antigens, which have been exploited as efficacious vaccine strategies in models of ovarian [45], metastatic melanoma [46, 47] and pancreatic [48] cancers. The latter study was recently expanded to a phase I clinical trial (NCI-2010-01868 and NCI-2013-02238) exploring safety and tolerability for a pancreatic cancer CSC vaccine [49]. These studies show selective depletion of CSCs in tumours after pulsing DCs with CSC-derived material, indicating that a specific T cell response can be generated against CSCs in vivo and is efficacious in reducing tumour burden. In addition to cytotoxic T cells, NK cells have also been shown to have preferential killing ability towards CSCs, which upregulate the NK cell recognition ligands MICA/B as well as the death receptors FAS and DR5 [50].

Immunotherapy for Dormant Tumours

While it remains unclear whether dormant tumour cells may share similar immune-modulatory properties as CSCs, if they do, these reports suggest that common immunotherapeutic strategies may target dormant tumour cells [51–53]. Certainly, reports of high expression of PD-L1 on CSCs [54] suggests that these cells could be targets of monoclonal antibody immunotherapies directed against the PD-1/PD-L1 checkpoint pathway, such as nivolumab, pembrolizumab and atezolizumab [55–57]. Across many solid tumour types, defining checkpoint molecule expression and immune cells in the tumour and circulation predict response to immunotherapy and/ or correlate with prognosis. Multiple studies have shown greater objective responses to immunotherapies where targets, such as PD-L1, are present on tumour [58–62] cells. However, this is not an absolute requirement for response, and mounting evidence indicates the importance of tumour infiltrating lymphocytes (TIL) and circulating immune cell correlates in disease progression. For example, expression of PD-L1/PD-1 by circulating innate immune and T cells is a prognostic indicator for glioblastoma, pancreatic, hepatocellular and lung cancer [5, 6, 8, 9] as well as responses to checkpoint blockade with Ipilimumab [7]. Furthermore, in a study that looked at seven different tumour types, PD-L1[+] TILs were strongly associated with response to anti-PD-L1 therapy [63]. Importantly however, these studies have all been conducted using sections from primary, or relapsed metastatic tumours, which cannot be defined as dormant tumours. It thus remains highly unclear whether in a dormant setting, the presence of checkpoint molecules on tumour or immune cells are similarly prognostic.

By definition, dormant tumour cells are in equilibrium with the immune response; therefore a rationally designed immunotherapeutic strategy against dormant tumours must either initiate their exit from dormancy or specifically target the unique elements of dormant tumours. Classical interventions like chemotherapy or radiation may provide the initial trigger causing tumour cells to exit the dormant phase, after which an immune response can be mounted. For example, dendritic cells increase tumour antigen presentation at low chemotherapeutic doses [64] and the abscopal effect that is observed after radiotherapy to localized tumours has been attributed to immune-mediated clearance of distant metastases [65, 66]. Chemotherapy can also have direct effects on immune cells; immunogenic drugs, such as oxaliplatin combined with cyclophosphamide, increase sensitivity of tumours to checkpoint blockade therapy [67]. Similarly, epigenetic targeting therapies are associated with upregulation of immune checkpoints. In leukemia [68, 69] and NSCLC [70], treatment with the DNA hypomethylating agent Azacitidine increases PD-1 or PD-L1 promoter demethylation and their expression. Importantly, the exit from dormancy initiated by chemo or radiotherapy is most likely associated with the release of neoantigens and other damage-associated molecules from the tumour that trigger immune responses [71]. The importance of increasing immunogenicity of tumours is underscored by the widespread efforts to design anti-cancer vaccines [72–74]. These may be especially relevant in the context of more dormant tumours such as Prostate, for which the first and only cancer vaccine has been approved [75, 76].

Thus, combining immunotherapies with therapies such as chemotherapies, radiation or epigenetic therapies, that alter the neo-antigen repertoire or checkpoint expression pattern of dormant tumour cells, is a potentially promising treatment strategy.

Ultimately, anticancer immunity is a prerequisite for the successful outcome of conventional cancer therapies [65, 66, 77–79]. While the immune response against tumour associated antigens can be elicited by either the innate or adaptive immune systems [78, 80], the goal of active immunotherapy is to achieve anti-tumour immunity. Therefore, apart from designing comprehensive studies related to phenotyping and genotyping of dormant tumours, it is important to consider therapies or combinatorial therapies that are designed for the specific dormant cancer phenotype.

References

1. Dunn GP, Bruce AT, Ikeda H, Old LJ, Schreiber RD (2002) Cancer immunoediting: from immunosurveillance to tumor escape. Nat Immunol 3(11):991–998
2. Ikeda H, Old LJ, Schreiber RD (2002) The roles of IFNγ in protection against tumor development and cancer immunoediting. Cytokine Growth Factor Rev 13(2):95–109

3. Kim JM, Chen DS (2016) Immune escape to PD-L1/PD-1 blockade: seven steps to success (or failure). Ann Oncol 27(8):1492–1504

4. Chen Daniel S, Mellman I (2013) Oncology meets immunology: the cancer-immunity cycle. Immunity 39(1):1–10

5. Basso D, Fogar P, Falconi M, Fadi E, Sperti C, Frasson C et al (2013) Pancreatic tumors and immature immunosuppressive myeloid cells in blood and spleen: role of inhibitory co-stimulatory molecules PDL1 and CTLA4. An in vivo and in vitro study. PLoS One 8(1):e54824. PubMed PMID: PMC3554636

6. Bloch O, Crane CA, Kaur R, Safaee M, Rutkowski MJ, Parsa AT (2013) Gliomas promote immunosuppression through induction of B7-H1 expression in tumor-associated macrophages. Clin Cancer Res 19(12):3165–3175

7. Tarhini AA, Edington H, Butterfield LH, Lin Y, Shuai Y, Tawbi H et al (2014) Immune monitoring of the circulation and the tumor microenvironment in patients with regionally advanced melanoma receiving neoadjuvant ipilimumab. PLoS One 9(2):e87705. PubMed PMID: PMC3912016

8. Waki K, Yamada T, Yoshiyama K, Terazaki Y, Sakamoto S, Matsueda S et al (2014) PD-1 expression on peripheral blood T-cell subsets correlates with prognosis in non-small cell lung cancer. Cancer Sci 105(10):1229–1235. PubMed PMID: PMC4462362

9. Zeng Z, Shi F, Zhou L, Zhang M-N, Chen Y, Chang X-J et al (2011) Upregulation of circulating PD-L1/PD-1 is associated with poor post-cryoablation prognosis in patients with HBV-related hepatocellular carcinoma. PLoS One 6(9):e23621. PubMed PMID: PMC3164659

10. Romero I, Garrido F, Garcia-Lora AM (2014) Metastases in immune-mediated dormancy: a new opportunity for targeting cancer. Cancer Res 74(23):6750–6757

11. Pitt Jonathan M, Vétizou M, Daillère R, Roberti María P, Yamazaki T, Routy B et al (2016) Resistance mechanisms to immune-checkpoint blockade in cancer: tumor-intrinsic and -extrinsic factors. Immunity 44(6):1255–1269

12. Serafini P, Carbley R, Noonan KA, Tan G, Bronte V, Borrello I (2004) High-dose granulocyte-macrophage colony-stimulating factor-producing vaccines impair the immune response through the recruitment of myeloid suppressor cells. Cancer Res 64(17):6337–6343

13. Chen W, Jin W, Hardegen N, Lei K-J, Li L, Marinos N et al (2003) Conversion of peripheral CD4(+)CD25(−) naive T cells to CD4(+)CD25(+) regulatory T cells by TGF-β induction of transcription factor Foxp3. J Exp Med 198(12):1875–1886. PubMed PMID: PMC2194145

14. Mellor AL, Munn DH (2004) Ido expression by dendritic cells: tolerance and tryptophan catabolism. Nat Rev Immunol 4(10):762–774

15. Lindau D, Gielen P, Kroesen M, Wesseling P, Adema GJ (2013) The immunosuppressive tumour network: myeloid-derived suppressor cells, regulatory T cells and natural killer T cells. Immunology 138(2):105–115. PubMed PMID: PMC3575763

16. Napolitano M, D'Alterio C, Cardone E, Trotta AM, Pecori B, Rega D et al (2015) Peripheral myeloid-derived suppressor and T regulatory PD-1 positive cells predict response to neoadjuvant short-course radiotherapy in rectal cancer patients. Oncotarget 6(10):8261–8270. PubMed PMID: PMC4480750

17. Schlecker E, Stojanovic A, Eisen C, Quack C, Falk CS, Umansky V et al (2012) Tumor-infiltrating monocytic myeloid-derived suppressor cells mediate CCR5-dependent recruitment of regulatory T cells favoring tumor growth. J Immunol 189(12):5602–5611

18. Zhang B, Wang Z, Wu L, Zhang M, Li W, Ding J et al (2013) Circulating and tumor-infiltrating myeloid-derived suppressor cells in patients with colorectal carcinoma. PLoS One 8(2):e57114. PubMed PMID: PMC3577767

19. Engels EA, Pfeiffer RM, Fraumeni JF et al (2011) Spectrum of cancer risk among us solid organ transplant recipients. JAMA 306(17):1891–1901

20. Dahlke E, Murray CA, Kitchen J, Chan A-W (2014) Systematic review of melanoma incidence and prognosis in solid organ transplant recipients. Transpl Res 3(1):10

21. Sharma P, Allison JP (2015) The future of immune checkpoint therapy. Science 348(6230):56

22. Fridman WH, Pagès F, Sautès-Fridman C, Galon J (2012) The immune contexture in human tumours: impact on clinical outcome. Nat Rev Cancer 12(4):298–306

23. Kroemer G, Senovilla L, Galluzzi L, Andre F, Zitvogel L (2015) Natural and therapy-induced immunosurveillance in breast cancer. Nat Med 21(10):1128–1138
24. Quesnel B (2013) Tumor dormancy: long-term survival in a hostile environment. In: Enderling H, Almog N, Hlatky L (eds) Systems biology of tumor dormancy. Springer, New York, pp 181–200
25. Sosa MS, Bragado P, Aguirre-Ghiso JA (2014) Mechanisms of disseminated cancer cell dormancy: an awakening field. Nat Rev Cancer 14(9):611–622
26. Ruppender NS, Morrissey C, Lange PH, Vessella RL (2013) Dormancy in solid tumors: implications for prostate cancer. Cancer Metastasis Rev 32(3–4):501–509. doi:10.1007/s10555-013-9422-z. PubMed PMID: PMC3796576
27. Gonzalez-Angulo AM, Morales-Vasquez F, Hortobagyi GN (2007) Overview of resistance to systemic therapy in patients with breast cancer. In: Yu D, Hung M-C (eds) Breast cancer chemosensitivity. Springer, New York, pp 1–22
28. Faries MB, Steen S, Ye X, Sim M, Morton DL (2013) Late recurrence in melanoma: clinical implications of lost dormancy. J Am Coll Surg 217(1):27–34. PubMed PMID: PMC3731060
29. Davis TA, Maloney DG, Czerwinski DK, Liles T-M, Levy R (1998) Anti-idiotype antibodies can induce long-term complete remissions in non-Hodgkin's lymphoma without eradicating the malignant clone. Blood 92(4):1184–1190
30. Beger HG, Rau B, Gansauge F, Leder G, Schwarz M, Poch B (2008) Pancreatic cancer—low survival rates. Dtsch Ärztebl Int 105(14):255–262. PubMed PMID: PMC2696777
31. Walid MS (2008) Prognostic factors for long-term survival after glioblastoma. Perm J 12(4):45–48. PubMed PMID: PMC3037140
32. Yang P (2009) Epidemiology of lung cancer prognosis: quantity and quality of life. Methods Mol Biol (Clifton, NJ) 471:469–486. PubMed PMID: PMC2941142
33. D'Amico TA (2007) Outcomes after surgery for esophageal cancer. Gastrointest Cancer Res 1(5):188–196. PubMed PMID: PMC2632530
34. Kleffel S, Schatton T (2013) Tumor dormancy and cancer stem cells: two sides of the same coin? In: Enderling H, Almog N, Hlatky L (eds) Systems biology of tumor dormancy. Springer, New York, pp 145–179
35. Plaks V, Kong N, Werb Z (2015) The cancer stem cell niche: how essential is the niche in regulating stemness of tumor cells? Cell Stem Cell 16(3):225–238
36. Zhang H, Lu H, Xiang L, Bullen JW, Zhang C, Samanta D et al (2015) HIF-1 regulates CD47 expression in breast cancer cells to promote evasion of phagocytosis and maintenance of cancer stem cells. Proc Natl Acad Sci U S A 112(45):E6215–E6E23. PubMed PMID: PMC4653179
37. Lee Y, Sunwoo J (2014) PD-L1 is preferentially expressed on CD44+ tumor-initiating cells in head and neck squamous cell carcinoma. J Immunother Cancer 2(Suppl 3):P270. PubMed PMID: PMC4292581
38. Jinushi M (2014) Role of cancer stem cell-associated inflammation in creating pro-inflammatory tumorigenic microenvironments. Oncoimmunology 3:e28862. PubMed PMID: PMC4091611
39. Bishop JL, Davies A, Ketola K, Zoubeidi A (2015) Regulation of tumor cell plasticity by the androgen receptor in prostate cancer. Endocr Relat Cancer 22(3):R165–R182
40. Bishop JL, Sio A, Angeles A, Roberts ME, Azad AA, Chi KN et al (2015) PD-L1 is highly expressed in enzalutamide resistant prostate cancer. Oncotarget 6(1):234–242. PubMed PMID: PMC4381591
41. Lee Y, Shin JH, Longmire M, Wang H, Kohrt HE, Chang HY et al (2016) CD44+ cells in head and neck squamous cell carcinoma suppress T-cell–mediated immunity by selective constitutive and inducible expression of PD-L1. Clin Cancer Res 22(14):3571–3581
42. Zhi Y, Mou Z, Chen J, He Y, Dong H, Fu X et al (2015) B7H1 expression and epithelial-to-mesenchymal transition phenotypes on colorectal cancer stem-like cells. PLoS One 10(8):e0135528. PubMed PMID: PMC4540313
43. Schatton T, Schütte U, Frank NY, Zhan Q, Hoerning A, Robles SC et al (2010) Modulation of t cell activation by malignant melanoma initiating cells. Cancer Res 70(2):697–708. PubMed PMID: PMC2883769

44. Grange C, Tapparo M, Tritta S, Deregibus MC, Battaglia A, Gontero P et al (2015) Role of HLA-G and extracellular vesicles in renal cancer stem cell-induced inhibition of dendritic cell differentiation. BMC Cancer 15:1009. PubMed PMID: PMC4690241

45. Wu D, Wang J, Cai Y, Ren M, Zhang Y, Shi F et al (2015) Effect of targeted ovarian cancer immunotherapy using ovarian cancer stem cell vaccine. J Ovarian Res 8:68. PubMed PMID: PMC4620009

46. Dashti A, Ebrahimi M, Hadjati J, Memarnejadian A, Moazzeni SM (2016) Dendritic cell based immunotherapy using tumor stem cells mediates potent antitumor immune responses. Cancer Lett 374(1):175–185

47. Hu Y, Lu L, Xia Y, Chen X, Chang AE, Hollingsworth RE et al (2016) Therapeutic efficacy of cancer stem cell vaccines in the adjuvant setting. Cancer Res 76(16):4661–4672

48. Xu Q, Liu G, Yuan X, Xu M, Wang H, Ji J et al (2009) Antigen-specific T-cell response from dendritic cell vaccination using cancer stem-like cell-associated antigens. Stem Cells 27(8):1734–1740

49. Lin M, Yuan Y-Y, Liu S-P, Shi J-J, Long X-A, Niu L-Z et al (2015) Prospective study of the safety and efficacy of a pancreatic cancer stem cell vaccine. J Cancer Res Clin Oncol 141(10):1827–1833

50. Ames E, Canter RJ, Grossenbacher SK, Mac S, Chen M, Smith RC et al (2015) NK cells preferentially target tumor cells with a cancer stem cell phenotype. J Immunol 195(8):4010–4019. PubMed PMID: PMC4781667

51. Canter RJ, Grossenbacher SK, Ames E, Murphy WJ (2016) Immune targeting of cancer stem cells in gastrointestinal oncology. J Gastrointest Oncol 7(Suppl 1):S1–S10. PubMed PMID: PMC4783622

52. Codony-Servat J, Rosell R (2015) Cancer stem cells and immunoresistance: clinical implications and solutions. Transl Lung Cancer Res 4(6):689–703. PubMed PMID: PMC4700228

53. Maccalli C, Volontè A, Cimminiello C, Parmiani G (2014) Immunology of cancer stem cells in solid tumours. A review. Eur J Cancer 50(3):649–655

54. Hirohashi Y, Torigoe T, Tsukahara T, Kanaseki T, Kochin V, Sato N (2016) Immune responses to human cancer stem-like cells/cancer-initiating cells. Cancer Sci 107(1):12–17. PubMed PMID: PMC4724814

55. Jazirehi AR, Lim A, Dinh T (2016) PD-1 inhibition and treatment of advanced melanoma-role of pembrolizumab. Am J Cancer Res 6(10):2117–2128. PubMed PMID: PMC5088280

56. Rosenberg JE, Hoffman-Censits J, Powles T, van der Heijden MS, Balar AV, Necchi A et al (2016) Atezolizumab in patients with locally advanced and metastatic urothelial carcinoma who have progressed following treatment with platinum-based chemotherapy: a single-arm, multicentre, phase 2 trial. Lancet 387(10031):1909–1920

57. Sundar R, Cho B-C, Brahmer JR, Soo RA (2015) Nivolumab in NSCLC: latest evidence and clinical potential. Ther Adv Med Oncol 7(2):85–96. PubMed PMID: PMC4346216

58. Brahmer JR, Drake CG, Wollner I, Powderly JD, Picus J, Sharfman WH et al (2010) Phase I study of single-agent anti-programmed death-1 (MDX-1106) in refractory solid tumors: safety, clinical activity, pharmacodynamics, and immunologic correlates. J Clin Oncol 28(19):3167–3175. PubMed PMID: PMC4834717

59. Taube JM, Klein A, Brahmer JR, Xu H, Pan X, Kim JH et al (2014) Association of PD-1, PD-1 ligands, and other features of the tumor immune microenvironment with response to anti-PD-1 therapy. Clin Cancer Res 20(19):5064–5074. PubMed PMID: PMC4185001

60. Topalian SL, Hodi FS, Brahmer JR, Gettinger SN, Smith DC, McDermott DF et al (2012) Safety, activity, and immune correlates of anti-PD-1 antibody in cancer. N Engl J Med 366(26):2443–2454. PubMed PMID: PMC3544539

61. Weber JS, Kudchadkar RR, Yu B, Gallenstein D, Horak CE, Inzunza HD et al (2013) Safety, efficacy, and biomarkers of nivolumab with vaccine in ipilimumab-refractory or -naive melanoma. J Clin Oncol 31(34):4311–4318. PubMed PMID: PMC3837092

62. Wolchok JD, Kluger H, Callahan MK, Postow MA, Rizvi NA, Lesokhin AM et al (2013) Nivolumab plus ipilimumab in advanced melanoma. N Engl J Med 369(2):122–133. PubMed PMID: 23724867

63. Herbst RS, Soria J-C, Kowanetz M, Fine GD, Hamid O, Gordon MS et al (2014) Predictive correlates of response to the anti-PD-L1 antibody MPDL3280A in cancer patients. Nature 515(7528):563–567
64. Shurin GV, Tourkova IL, Kaneno R, Shurin MR (2009) Chemotherapeutic agents in noncytotoxic concentrations increase antigen presentation by dendritic cells via an IL-12-dependent mechanism. J Immunol 183(1):137–144. PubMed PMID: PMC4005417
65. Hamanishi J, Mandai M, Iwasaki M, Okazaki T, Tanaka Y, Yamaguchi K et al (2007) Programmed cell death 1 ligand 1 and tumor-infiltrating CD8(+) T lymphocytes are prognostic factors of human ovarian cancer. Proc Natl Acad Sci U S A 104(9):3360–3365. PubMed PMID: PMC1805580
66. Radvanyi L (2013) Immunotherapy exposes cancer stem cell resistance and a new synthetic lethality. Mol Therapy 21(8):1472–1474. PubMed PMID: PMC3740219
67. Pfirschke C, Engblom C, Rickelt S, Cortez-Retamozo V, Garris C, Pucci F et al (2016) Immunogenic chemotherapy sensitizes tumors to checkpoint blockade therapy. Immunity 44(2):343–354
68. Ørskov AD, Treppendahl MB, Skovbo A, Holm MS, Friis LS, Hokland M et al (2015) Hypomethylation and up-regulation of PD-1 in T cells by azacytidine in MDS/AML patients: a rationale for combined targeting of PD-1 and DNA methylation. Oncotarget 6(11):9612–9626
69. Yang H, Bueso-Ramos C, DiNardo C, Estecio MR, Davanlou M, Geng QR et al (2014) Expression of PD-L1, PD-L2, PD-1 and CTLA4 in myelodysplastic syndromes is enhanced by treatment with hypomethylating agents. Leukemia 28(6):1280–1288
70. Wrangle J, Wang W, Koch A, Easwaran H, Mohammad HP, Pan X et al (2013) Alterations of immune response of non-small cell lung cancer with Azacytidine. Oncotarget 4(11):2067–2079
71. Ma Y, Conforti R, Aymeric L, Locher C, Kepp O, Kroemer G et al (2011) How to improve the immunogenicity of chemotherapy and radiotherapy. Cancer Metastasis Rev 30(1):71–82
72. Kumai T, Kobayashi H, Harabuchi Y, Celis E (2017) Peptide vaccines in cancer—old concept revisited. Curr Opin Immunol 45:1–7
73. Thomas S, Prendergast GC (2016) Cancer vaccines: a brief overview. In: Thomas S (ed) Vaccine design: methods and protocols: vol 1: vaccines for human diseases. Springer, New York, pp 755–761
74. Wong KK, Li WA, Mooney DJ, Dranoff G (2016) Chapter five—advances in therapeutic cancer vaccines. In: Robert DS (ed) Advances in immunology, vol 130. Academic, New York, pp 191–249
75. Gulley JL, Mulders P, Albers P, Banchereau J, Bolla M, Pantel K et al (2016) Perspectives on sipuleucel-T: its role in the prostate cancer treatment paradigm. Oncoimmunology 5(4):e1107698. PubMed PMID: PMC4839373
76. Tse BW-C, Jovanovic L, Nelson CC, de Souza P, Power CA, Russell PJ (2014) From bench to bedside: immunotherapy for prostate cancer. Biomed Res Int 2014:981434. PubMed PMID: PMC4168152
77. Arenas-Ramirez N, Zou C, Popp S, Zingg D, Brannetti B, Wirth E et al (2016) Improved cancer immunotherapy by a CD25-mimobody conferring selectivity to human interleukin-2. Sci Transl Med 8(367):367ra166–367ra166
78. Spurrell EL, Lockley M (2014) Adaptive immunity in cancer immunology and therapeutics. ecancermedicalscience 8:441. PubMed PMID: PMC4096025
79. Yoshimoto T, Chiba Y, Furusawa J-I, Xu M, Tsunoda R, Higuchi K et al (2015) Potential clinical application of interleukin-27 as an antitumor agent. Cancer Sci 106(9):1103–1110. PubMed PMID: PMC4582978
80. Liu Y, Zeng G (2012) Cancer and innate immune system interactions: translational potentials for cancer immunotherapy. J Immunother 35(4):299–308. PubMed PMID: PMC3331796

Thermodynamics and Cancer Dormancy: A Perspective

Edward A. Rietman and Jack A. Tuszynski

Abstract In this review we elaborate on the hypothesis that concepts adapted from statistical thermodynamics, such as entropy and Gibbs free energy, can provide very powerful quantitative measures when applied to cancer research, in particular to cancer dormancy. We discuss how on all size scales of biological organization hierarchy from DNA to tissue and organ representation, cancer progression can be correlated with these thermodynamic measures. Significant diagnostic, prognostic and therapeutic implications of these new organizing principles are presented.

Keywords Cancer • Statistical thermodynamics • Entropy • Information • Gibbs free energy • Dormancy

Introduction: Entropy and Information

Physics has evolved over the past 400 years from an empirical science to a fundamental basis of human knowledge. This took place as a result of several revolutions in our understanding of nature ushered by the discovery of new organizing principles called laws of physics. To name some of them, Newton's laws of mechanics, Maxwell's theory of electromagnetism, quantum mechanics as embodied by Schrödinger's, Heisenberg's and Dirac's equations for the time-dependence of states and theory representations and, finally, Einstein's theories or special and general relativity [1], can be viewed as major framework for our description of the universe. All of these mathematical representations of physical reality changed the way we understand, interpret and shape the world around us. No less dramatic, albeit less known to the general public, was the introduction of the laws of

E.A. Rietman (✉)
Computer Science Department, University of Massachusetts, Amherst, MA, USA
e-mail: erietman@umass.edu

J.A. Tuszynski
Department of Oncology, University of Alberta, Edmonton, AB, Canada, T6G 1Z2

Department of Physics, University of Alberta, Edmonton, AB, Canada, T6G 1Z2
e-mail: jackt@ualberta.ca

© Springer International Publishing AG 2017
Y. Wang, F. Crea (eds.), *Tumor Dormancy and Recurrence*, Cancer Drug Discovery and Development, DOI 10.1007/978-3-319-59242-8_5

thermodynamics into the physics vocabulary by Ludwig Boltzmann [2]. Boltzmann's concept of entropy, despite being one of the most powerful ideas in physics, was fiercely resisted by his contemporaries. Yet, Boltzmann's finding that all closed physical systems tend to a state of maximum entropy is a very powerful observation, which is yet to be contradicted by any experimental evidence, and which has found numerous applications not only in physics, but also in fields as diverse as sociology, financial markets and drug discovery [3].

The present expansion of biology is reminiscent of the state of physics at the turn of the nineteenth and twentieth century. Reams of data about physical systems are being collected, but there is a dire lack of organizing principles or major conceptual framework. Most of the research in the area of life sciences is advanced on the basis of *ad hoc* hypotheses and their empirical validation. Molecular biology and sister fields such as genetics, cell biology and others continue to collect masses of real-life data, but the data can only be visualized or organized computationally. The lack of organizing principles leaves researchers at the mercy of computational tools. In 1944 in his book entitled "What is Life", Erwin Schrödinger, a Nobel-Prize winning physicist, exposed some of the main challenges found in biology from physics point of view [4]. He implied for example that the reduction of entropy in living systems seems to contradict the second law of thermodynamics. The answer to this conundrum lies not only in physics but also in information science because entropy is negatively correlated with information as defined by the great computer scientist Claude Shannon [5].

In thermodynamics, entropy (denoted commonly by the symbol S) is a measure of the number of microscopic configurations that correspond to realization of a thermodynamic system in a state specified by certain macroscopic variables. For example, gas in a container with known volume, pressure, and temperature could have an enormous number of possible configurations of the individual gas molecules, each of which may be regarded as random. Hence, entropy can be understood as a measure of molecular disorder within a macroscopic system. The second law of thermodynamics states that an isolated system's entropy never decreases. Thermodynamic systems spontaneously evolve towards thermodynamic equilibrium, which can be mathematically proven to be the state with maximum entropy. Non-isolated systems, i.e. those that interact with their environment, may reduce their entropy, provided their environment's entropy increases by at least the same amount. Since entropy is a thermodynamic state function, the change in entropy of a system is determined by its initial and final states. This applies whether the process is reversible or irreversible. However, irreversible processes increase the combined entropy of the system and its environment while entropy is conserved in reversible processes. Entropy is an extensive thermodynamic property which means that it is additive, so that the entropy of a system composed of a number of subsystems is the sum of their respective subsystem entropies. This is very useful, especially in the context of biological systems, which by definition are heterogeneous and hierarchical.

In statistical thermodynamics the most general mathematical formula for the thermodynamic entropy S of a thermodynamic system is the so-called Gibbs entropy introduced by J. Willard Gibbs in 1878 as

$$S = -k_B \sum p_i \ln p_i \tag{1}$$

where k_B is the Boltzmann constant, and p_i is the probability of a particular micro-state denoted by the subscript i. The connection between thermodynamics and information theory was first made by Ludwig Boltzmann and expressed by his famous equation expressing entropy as

$$S = k_B \ln\left(W\right) \tag{2}$$

where S corresponds to the thermodynamic entropy of a particular macrostate (defined by macroscopic thermodynamic parameters such as temperature, volume, energy, etc.), W is the number of microstates that can yield the given macrostate. It is assumed that each microstate is equally likely, so that the probability of a given microstate is $p_i = 1/W$. When these probabilities are substituted into the above expression for the Gibbs entropy, Boltzmann's equation results. In information theoretic terms, the information entropy of a system is the amount of "missing" information needed to determine a microstate, given the macrostate. The average amount of information, I, that is gained with every event is equal to the opposite of entropy (negentropy), i.e.:

$$\sum_i p_i \log \frac{1}{p_i}. \tag{3}$$

In the modern microscopic interpretation of entropy in statistical mechanics, entropy is the amount of additional information needed to specify the exact physical state of a system, given its thermodynamic description. Understanding the role of thermodynamic entropy in various processes requires an understanding of how and why that information changes as the system evolves from its initial to its final condition. It is often said that entropy is an expression of the disorder, or randomness of a system, or of our lack of information about it. The second law of thermodynamics is often seen as an expression of the fundamental postulate of statistical mechanics through the modern definition of entropy. A tendency towards equilibrium in statistical systems of many particles can be viewed as simply a natural evolution to the most probable situation. In isolated systems this means maximum entropy under constraints. In interacting systems, this means a minimum of an appropriate thermodynamic potential such as the Gibbs free energy. These simple statements laid the foundations of numerous applications of statistical mechanics in physics and beyond and form a conceptual framework that allows us to think about immensely complex systems of many particles within a single organizing principle.

Complexity of Cancer

The need to organize biological information is particularly acute in cancer research. Despite vast amounts of accumulated and emerging genetic, molecular, cellular, histological and epidemiological information, and despite intense efforts to identify predisposing factors (e.g. carcinogens, reactive oxidants, genetic/family history), cancer remains an enormous and in general unresolved enigma. Malignant cells have selectively evolved to divide and multiply at the expense of the host. They evade programmed cell death (apoptosis), and further enhance proliferative potential. As they invade surrounding tissues and ablate tissue architecture, they disturb normal paracrine systems and stimulate coagulation, inflammation and formation of blood vessels (angiogenesis). Because terminal cell differentiation (cell phenotype) depends on tissue stimuli, the process is disturbed, leading to lack of cell maturation, de-differentiation, or even trans-differentiation in the form of epithelial to mesenchymal transformation [6, 7].

In the early twentieth century German biologist Theodor Boveri observed cell division ("mitosis") in normal and cancerous cells [8]. Boveri noticed that while normal cells exhibited symmetrical, bipolar division of chromosomes into two equivalent mirror-like allocations, cancer cells were different. Cancer cells had higher frequency of imbalanced divisions of chromosomes, with asymmetrical and multipolar imbalanced ("aneuploid") distributions. Boveri had suggested that the abnormal distribution of chromosomes and genes was caused by aberrant mitosis, and reasoned that even though most abnormal distributions would be non-viable, some would lead to viable cells with proliferative advantage. Furthermore, because imbalance in chromosomal distribution could not result in recurrent, identifiable division pattern, aneuploidy would change with each subsequent generation leading to what is now known as "genomic instability". In the past, most scientists assumed that the abnormal distributions of chromosomes were a result, rather than a cause of malignant transformation and that cancer originated from intrinsic mutational changes [9]. While in retrospect, genomic instability appears to be a logical consequence of abnormal mitosis, the belief that cancer resulted from randomly accumulated genetic mutations has become a widely accepted standard, a "dogma".

As DNA and genetics became better understood and took a prominent position in life sciences, the hypothesis that cancer is the result of cumulative mutations became entrenched and a somewhat simplistic model of sequential genetic mutations facilitating an accelerated somatic cell evolution into a fast proliferating, drug resistant cancer clone emerged. The theory was supported by the observation that many cancers arose from persistently proliferating tissues such as hepatocellular carcinoma in chronic viral hepatitis, or esophageal cancer caused by Barrett's esophagus. This was further reinforced by publications documenting that genetic alterations are considerably more abundant in cancer cells than previously expected, with 11,000 genomic events per (colon) carcinoma cell [10].

The cancer cell-specific alterations in the DNA, whether spontaneous or induced by carcinogens, were thought to lead to changes in the respective proteins encoded by cancer-related genes. Two types of cancer-related genes were identified: the first included tumor suppressor genes, which lead to cancer predisposition, and the second were oncogenes, which directly induce malignant transformation. Tumor suppressor genes can work in many ways; they can remove an inhibitor on a proliferative pathway (e.g. PTEN), create chromosomal instability (e.g. p53), or cause an abnormal DNA repair (RB)—in each case a second mutation (a "second hit") is needed for cancer to develop. Oncogenes, in contrast, are genomic alterations resulting in over-expression or constitutional activation of genes that stimulate growth and cell division, or which inhibit apoptosis.

But the oncogene/tumor suppressor gene theory has failed to fully explain carcinogenesis or cancer progression. In particular, the linear cancer progression model has failed to describe the fact that cancer progression is not a continuous incremental process. In fact, cancer cells can plastically stop their proliferation to adapt to challenging environments such as those posed by toxicity due to pharmacological agents and then resume the proliferation after years or they can trigger metastases to find a suitable niche environment for their successful proliferation. We have not been able to identify a set of gene mutations that would consistently correlate with cancer initiation, progression or dissemination. Even tumors with identical clinical and pathological diagnosis, exhibit unique and genetically distinct set of DNA alterations, that seem to be independent of the genetic make up of the host. This uniqueness is particularly evident in the tremendous genetic variability that occurs within a single individual tumor. As such, the concept of genomic instability, i.e. the continuous change in the tumor genetic makeup resulting from imbalance in chromosomal distribution with each subsequent mitotic cycle, is gaining acceptance.

The theory of sequential accumulation of random mutations leading to evolution of proliferative cancer clone, as well as the theory of imbalanced ("aneuploid") distribution of DNA leading to cancer, can be combined by considering that both theories must submit to the physical pressures occurring within the tumor microenvironment. Cancer evolution and the development of a heterogeneous, genetically and metabolically distinct tumor subclones may be a direct consequence of thermodynamic environment-dependent evolutionary pressures.

We argue here that thermodynamics is the driving force for cancer initiation, progression, dissemination and dormancy. While we recognize that mutations and *in situ* evolution plays a significant part, but those processes are driven by molecular, cellular, tissue and organ-specific thermodynamics. Thermodynamics dictates the possible. Kinetics dictates the probable.

In the following we address each scale in turn.

Molecular Scale

Some specific DNA factors are indeed related to genomic instability. These include unrepaired DNA damage, stalled DNA replication forks processed inappropriately by recombination enzymes, and defective telomeres, which protect ends of chromosomes. But again, inherent DNA mutation and sequelae—the "standard dogma"—don't explain the entire picture. Other approaches suggest that a combination of DNA defects and other problems are responsible for genomic instability and malignancy.

One approach is called "modified dogma" which revives an idea from 1974 by Loeb and colleagues [11] who noted that random mutations, on average, would affect only one gene per cell in a lifetime. Some other factor—carcinogen, reactive oxidants, malfunction in DNA duplication and repair machinery—is proposed to increase the incidence of random mutations [12]. Another approach is "early instability" [13] which suggests that master genes are critical to cell division—if they are mutated, mitosis is aberrant. But master genes are still merely proposals. Recently, Tomasetti and Vogelstein [14] presented epidemiological evidence which indicates that as many as 2/3 of all cancers are a result of random mutations since their incidence correlates with the frequency of cell divisions.

A cell is comprised of a large variety of molecules of different sizes, shapes and physical attributes interacting in a complex network. Whenever one, or more, of the molecular species lose the normally prevailing chemical equilibrium with their reaction partners, the resulting difference in chemical-potential alters the normally occurring chemical reactions within the network driving them in new directions. These new chemical, physical and energetic changes lead to evolutionary pressures enabling an entirely new set of mutational adaptations. It is well accepted in biology that a persistent change in intracellular environment leads to preservation/selection of a "protective" mutation. As an example of a chemical potential imbalance, a persistent abundance in extracellular glucose supply leads to preferential ATP production in the cytoplasmic fluid rather than the mitochondria [15]. This excess production in the cytoplasm results in a slight pH imbalance and the mitochondrial walls may breakdown. Since GTP is produced in the citric acid cycle in the mitochondria, this results in an inadequate supply of GTP—the end-cap for the microtubules (MT) in the cytoplasm. Insufficient numbers of end-caps for the MTs can result in mitotic catastrophe, or in aneuploidy and cancer [16].

One can therefore use the degree of entropy of established protein-protein interaction (PPI) networks to assess cancer risk and survival. Because the degree entropy of a PPI network is essentially a Boltzmann distribution, it is a thermodynamic observation. Breitkreutz et al. [17] found that the degree entropy of cancer PPI networks included in the Kyoto Encyclopedia of Genes (KEGG) inversely correlated with 5-year survival of cancer patients. Each cancer PPI network is characterized by a type of different entropy, but in all cases studied entropy of the network could be inversely correlated with 5-year survival. The observed degree entropy corresponded to the complexity of the molecular PPI network, and a mathematical elimination of proteins leading to decrease in network complexity could be correlated to improved survival rates [18].

Cellular Scale

Multiple mechanisms within a cell are responsible for maintaining cell integrity and function. A great example of these mechanisms is the production of ATP through oxidative phosphorylation in the mitochondria, which is responsible for providing energy to cells. Mitochondrial function is subject to strict temporal and spatial coordination, and thus a hub of dynamic instability. Variations in mitochondrial metabolism may be secondary to changes in cellular events such as glycolysis [19], Ca^{2+} influx [20], changes in membrane potential [21], or may be intrinsic [22] to mitochondria.

Carels et al. [23] have applied the concepts of entropy maximization in the context of different breast cancer cell lines. They extended it to develop a strategy for the optimized selection of protein targets for drug development against breast cancer as an example. By combining human interactome and transcriptome data from malignant and control cell lines they described and quantified the highly connected proteins in these PPI networks. They assumed that proteins that are most upregulated in malignant cell lines are suitable targets for chemotherapy with a decreased rate of undesirable side effects since normal cells express them to a much lower degree. The most connected proteins that act as protein network hubs in the signaling network have been identified. In addition to traditional drug targets such as EGFR, MAPK13 or HSP90, they found several proteins, not generally targeted by drug treatments, which might justify the extension of existing formulation by addition of inhibitors designed against these proteins with the consequence of improving therapeutic outcomes. Their results reveal GABARAPL1 and GAPDH as hubs in BT-20 cells (triple negative breast cancer). Another class of targets is the group of genes involved in cell signaling and cell communication such as membrane proteins, HER2 and 3 or EGFR, signal transduction proteins such as MYC, TK1, NPM, YWHAB, MCM7, EIF4A3, HDGF, GRB2, CHD3, PAK2, PA2G4, and transport proteins such as KPNA2. It is not surprising that in this work, control genes of the cell cycle or apoptosis were pinpointed such as MAPK13, HSP90AB1, MAGOH, CSNK2B, EEF1G, PDIA3, ICT1, SRPK1, and also those involved in the EMT process such as VIM, which play a major role in tumor development HSP90AB1 was found to be the only upregulated protein hub common to all cell breast cancer types in this study, which highlights the fact that the cancer subtypes share a core of proliferative signaling pathways common in breast cancers, but with many specificities.

The molecular alterations observed in breast cancer cell lines represent either driver events and/or driver pathways that are necessary for breast cancer development or progression. However, it is clear that signaling mechanisms of the luminal A, B and triple negative subtypes are different. Furthermore, the up- and downregulated networks predicted subtype-specific drug targets and possible compensation circuits between up- and downregulated genes. These results may have significant clinical implications in the personalized treatment of cancer patients allowing an objective approach to the recycling of the arsenal of available drugs to the specific case of each breast cancer given their distinct qualitative and quantitative molecular traits.

In a follow-up study, Carels et al. [24] investigated breast cancer cell lines and found that the entropy of their protein interaction networks is negatively correlated with their sensitivity to target-specific drugs of high potency. This sensitivity is defined as half cell growth inhibition (GI_{50}) with respect to drug administration. By contrast, they have found no correlation for drugs that are either of low potency or with no specific molecular targets (broadly cytotoxic). Interestingly, dormant cells are less sensitive to chemotherapy, which preferentially targets dividing cells and hence the plastic ability of cancer cells to alternate between dormant and proliferating states could be linked to increased cellular entropy. This is because increasing phenotypic phase space by adding dormancy is clearly an entropy-increasing outcome. As a result of the analysis above, all anti-cancer drugs have been divided into target-specific and generally cytotoxic according to the GI_{50} they produce in malignant cell lines. By extrapolation, these authors have predicted that the inactivation of the top-5 upregulated protein hubs by specific drugs may reduce the protein network entropy by ~2%, on average, which is expected to substantially increase the benefit of a personalized chemotherapeutic strategy for patient survival anticipating complete remission over a 5-year period of beyond.

Tissue Scale

The metabolic activity of mitochondria within a cell is the result of the coordination of several highly dynamic processes characterized by complex temporal patterns, which can display dynamic instability. An example of spatio-temporal coordination of mitochondrial metabolism in multi-cellular organisms *in situ* has been recently presented by Porat-Shliom et al. [25]. It is conceivable that pathological changes at a tissue level lead to disorganization and desynchronization, which in the context of metabolic oscillations, has a tendency to increase the entropy of the metabolic networks within the cancer tissue.

Rietman et al. [26] have described how to compute Gibbs free energy of PPI networks and discovered that it correlates with cancer stage. Their Gibbs free energy is a genuine thermodynamic measure computed from using the mRNA expression values for cancer patient tissues and overlaying that on the human PPI from BioGrid (http://thebiogrid.org).

One can calculate the Gibbs free energy from the chemical potential. For computing the Gibbs energy of a cell we use mRNA expression or RNAseq counts as a surrogate for protein concentration. Greenbaum et al. [27], Maier et al. [28], Kim et al. [29], Wihelm et al. [30], Liu et al. [31], Berretta and Moscato [32] all point to the use of RNA abundance as a measure of protein concentration. Once we have the concentration of each protein we can rescale the entire vector of transcriptome to be between 0 and 1. Essentially, this sets the lowest abundance RNA at 0 and the highest at 1.

These concentration values can now be used to compute the Gibbs free energy from knowledge of the PPI. For any given node in the PPI, i, the concentration is given by c_i and the free energy is:

$$G_i = c_i \ln \left[\frac{c_i}{\sum\limits_{j=i} c_j} \right] \quad (4)$$

where the sum is over all interaction neighbors j, including i. Carrying this out on several TCGA cancers, this can be first computed as indicated in the equation for the individual Gibbs free energy for a particular protein, but then it should be summed over all proteins to obtain the total Gibbs free energy of the network. This now represents an average of the Gibbs energy for that tissue sample from the biopsy. Table 1 (reproduced from Rietman et al. [33]) shows the Gibbs free energy correlating with 5-year survival.

Extending that work to look at Gibbs free energy of cancer stage using the same set of TCGA cancers and including two GEO datasets for prostate cancer GSE3933 [34] and GSE6099 [35] and a GEO dataset for liver cancer GSE6764 [36]. Processing the data for rescaling as described above, we can then calculate the Gibbs free energy on the individual cancer stage biopsy samples. The cancer stage, typically represented as a Roman numeral, was simply assigned an ordinal number. Then computing the Spearman's rho and Kendall tau as measures of fit we get the results shown in Table 1. The sign in front of the value for rho or tau indicates the slope of the fit. The tissue type dictates the slopes. It is not clear to us at this stage why these coefficients are positive in some types of cancer and negative in others. However, as can be readily seen, several of these cancers show very significantly linear correlation of Gibbs free energy to cancer stage. This is highly suggestive that the Gibbs free energy has captured a real thermodynamic measure of cancer stage.

Metabolic Entropy Increase in Cancer

Earlier we described how a glucose imbalance outside the cell will percolate, *via* the molecular network to result in a pH imbalance within the cell. Gillies et al. [37] have described an acidic extracellular environment of tumors. They go on to show that there is a similar imbalance in the pO_2 level and this can induce metastasis and invasion. The low pH and low pO_2 also results in resistance to therapies.

It is now generally accepted that tumors in general have an increased uptake of glucose. This high demand for glucose, even in the presence of adequate oxygen supply, has been referred to as the Warburg effect. The causes and advantages of increased glucose consumption of tumors have been extensively studied and reviewed in a number of publications [38–41]. These effects include protection from apoptosis, a resultant acidic microenvironment that gives cancer a proliferative

Table 1 Gibbs energy as a function of cancer stage for several cancer types [33]

TCGA name	Cancer type	Stages	Spearman's rho	Kendall tau	Number of samples in ordinal stage							Total
	Gibbs vs. cancer stage, from averages of Gibbs per stage				1	2	3	4	5	6	7	N
KIRC	Kidney renal clear cell	I, II, III, IV	−0.400	−0.333	38	13	14	5				70
BRCA	Breast invasive carcinoma	I, IIA, IIB, IIIA, IIIB, IIIC, IV	**0.762**	**0.571**	102	206	126	86	15	23	15	573
UCEC	Uterine corpus endometrial	I, II, III, IV	**−0.900**	**−0.800**	34	3	3	8				48
OV	Serous cystadenocarcinoma	I, II, IIIA, IIIB, IIIC, IV	**0.800**	**0.667**	16	28	30	387	78			539
COAD	Colon adenocarcinoma	I, II, III, IV	0.238	0.000	12	59	41	25				137
LUAD	Lung adenocarcinoma	I, II, III, IV	−0.100	0.000	82	34	34	4				154
LUSC	Lung squamous cell	I, II, III, IV	**0.800**	**0.600**	23	4	3	2				32
GEO	Liver (GSE6764)	See Rietman et al. [33]	**−0.999**	**−1.000**	9	10	10	7	18	17		71
GEO	Prostate (GSE3933, GSE6069)	See Rietman et al. [33]	**−1.000**	**−1.000**	8	12	79	5				104

Spearman's rho and Kendall's tau values >0.5 and <−0.5 indicate a strong correlation and are shown in bold advantage, as well as a mechanism to create most rapidly the biomass for tumor proliferation.

This increased consumption of glucose in cancer is associated with upregulated glycolysis, an anaerobic mechanism, which may lead to a significant energy burden to the cancer patient not previously integrated into resting energy expenditure (REE) estimates. REE is normally calculated by indirect calorimetry, which measures oxygen consumption, carbon dioxide production, and urea excretion. Complete aerobic metabolism is assumed [42], and thus anaerobic energy production is not accounted for. Therefore, the potentially large anaerobic energy usage of tumors is not factored into many calculations of the energy deficit of patients with cachexia, and thus late-stage cancer patients with large tumor burdens may have a much larger "hidden" energy deficit than commonly calculated.

Friesen et al. [43] have proposed a quantitative model incorporating a tumor's unique energy metabolism to describe how a tumor of sufficient mass will lead to an energetic burden, with glucose and glutamine consumption that could lead to the body's muscle wasting in order to fuel the tumor's energetic demands. The body may break down muscle preferentially as muscle breakdown is able to supply the additional need for glucose and glutamine by the tumor, causing cachexia. This muscle loss has the greatest impact on patients' quality of life and is associated with a poor survival outcome [44]. Furthermore, Friesen et al. [43] modeled this muscle and fat loss as a result of this energetic deficit based on our previous data on patients with advanced colorectal cancer and metastases in the liver, as well as previous studies monitoring glucose turnover in cachexic patients, and suggested specific treatment strategies based on this bioenergetic view of cancer cachexia. These authors have calculated that the energetic cost of a tumor may approach or exceed 1330 kcal/kg tumor/day when including the energetic cost of the tumor in feeding and fasting states and Cori cycling of lactate generated by the tumor. As tumors grow, this cost may eventually become prohibitive, and combined with reduced caloric intake as a result of the tumor, may lead to a catabolic, cachexic state. A corresponding picture of cancer development and progression through the stages ending with cachexia and death can be viewed as a continuous increase in metabolic entropy produced due to a highly inefficient glucose metabolism with a concomitant growth of the glycolytic rate as predicted by Warburg [45]. Additionally, going through cycles of growth and quiescence may be a clever evolutionary strategy to maintain the host alive so that the tumor can continue its parasitic relationship. This aspect can be simulated computationally by using a prey-predator type of mathematical modeling.

Organismal Scale

One of the most fundamental differences between animate and inanimate matter from the point of view of thermodynamics is that by definition the former exists in states that are far from thermodynamic equilibrium. Living systems survive only because there is a flux of matter and energy between them and their surroundings, and excess entropy transfer into their surroundings to compensate for the creation and maintenance of structural order (entropy reduction) and functional organization.

To apply thermodynamic concepts to cancer, we first need to determine what the relevant order and control parameters are. In the case of a transition from normal to cancer cells, the nature of the change taking place is one of molecular and cellular reorganization leading to a drastic elimination of various cell cycle check points and a simplification of the cell's functional program to one that seems to be aimed mainly at survival and proliferation, which could involve dormancy phases required for the establishment of distant metastases and for mounting effective drug resistance as an additional survival strategy under harsh environmental conditions. Although the trigger for cancer may reside at the molecular level (for example, the switching on of an oncogene, the disablement of a tumor suppressor gene or accumulated damage to DNA due to UV radiation or toxins), thermodynamic treatments are normally formulated in terms of *macroscopic* variables. Cells function as metabolic networks defined by a large ensemble of interacting enzymes within a substrate mediated by processes typically described using chemical kinetics transforming one metabolite into another. The existence of such networks supports the concept of describing cells in terms of aggregate variables; macroscopic parameters that are functions of the structure of the network and the biochemical interactions between the elements. In the case of cancer, it is not hard to identify relevant physical changes at the macroscopic level taking place in the affected organism. Indeed, it is mostly from such changes that cancer is diagnosed. These include the gross alterations in the structure, function, and organization of cells, and even to a certain extent the surrounding tissue microenvironment. For example, cancer cells display marked changes in viscoelastic properties, morphology, nuclear structure and chromatin architecture, and heterogeneity as well as dramatic changes in metabolism, pH values, and trans-membrane potentials. A qualitative description of the transformation from normal to cancer tissue using the concepts of phase transition that include order parameters, control parameters, Gibbs free energy and entropy and susceptibility has been provided by Davies et al. [46].

Fractal geometry is a powerful mathematical concepts that allows to quantify systems with self-similar properties by introducing the definition of fractal dimension. Furthermore, fractal dimension has been linked to both Shannon's entropy and Kolmogorov entropy, the latter describes the measure of chaoticity of a disordered system [47]. There are numerous studies measuring fractal dimension of cancer cells as well as cancer tissues. Very few studies, however, related Shannon entropy to diagnosis and prognosis of cancer [48]. This area still requires more quantitative and systematic studies, which could relate the fractal dimension of the tumor tissue with the corresponding entropy and further to the grade and stage of cancer.

Epidemiological Scale

Rietman et al. [33] describe the concept of Gibbs free energy on cancer stage, but go beyond that and apply a topological concept known as "filtration" [49] to produce what is known as a persistent homology from the energy landscape that the PPI with transcriptome represent. At any given threshold an energetic subnetwork is produced. Figure 1 is an example for oligodendroglioma (low-grade glioma). This is specific to this patient. Different patients will have different energetic persistent homology networks. If we now apply another topological concept known as the Betti number [18], essentially a count of the number of rings of four or more proteins, and find which node in the network when removed will drop the Betti number the most, as described by Rietman et al. [33] this becomes a suitable target for protein inhibition in treating this specific cancer patient.

We have already described correlations between molecular network thermodynamics and molecular network topology and cancer patient survival as demonstrated by Breitkreutz et al. [17] in great detail. Rietman et al. [33] show that Gibbs free energy correlates with 5-year survival. A corresponding quantitative analysis of the glycolytic switch rate and the resultant entropy increase correlating with a reduction in 5-year survival is conceptually straight-forward but to the best of the authors' knowledge has not been published yet.

Conclusions

In this paper we have brought evidence to support the statement that drug resistance and cancer progression (in terms of distinct stages) are associated with progressive changes in entropy and Gibbs free energy. Both phenomena have been linked to tumor dormancy, for example see [50]. A specific loss of p53 function as a "guardian of the genome" playing a central role in cell cycle maintenance is also linked to drug resistance and further to dormancy [51]. We also believe that dormancy fits into the organizing principle of entropy by enlarging the state space of the cancer cell and leading to increased heterogeneity. This is consistent with an entropy increase.

While the time dependence of the tumor growth is not explicitly built into this model, it appears that a monotonic representation of a continued progression of the cancer state into more malignant states is not supported by recent work on cancer modeling where competition between cancer and normal (including immune system cells) phenotypes leads to nonlinear behavior well described by a prey-predator set of differential eqs. [52]. The resultant oscillatory tumor growth pattern is known to produce "cycles" of quiescence and proliferation in most cancers. At present, it is not clear how time dependence in deterministic models of this type can be connected to entropy maximization without coupling the two subsystems (normal and malignant) in a dynamic interaction with opposite tendencies, i.e. the normal tissue

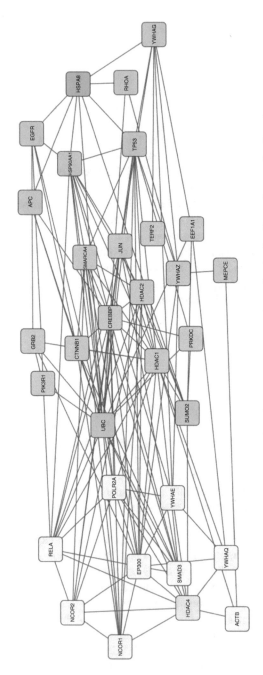

Fig. 1 A characteristic protein-protein interaction network for a patient diagnosed with a oligodendroglioma (low-grade glioma)

striving for entropy minimization under spatial and energetic constraints and tumor cells maximizing entropy. A mathematical description of this type of process is still lacking.

A war on cancer was boldly declared by US President Richard Nixon over 40 years ago and close to a trillion dollars was spent on cancer research since then. While incremental progress can be claimed on several fronts including advances in targeted chemotherapy, radiation tomotherapy and more accurate diagnostic tools, we are still almost clueless regarding the molecular-level causes of cancer and hence clinical outcomes have been far from impressive. Many of the cancer chemotherapy drugs are very expensive, provide modest clinical improvements and have significant negative side effects. We believe what is needed to make serious progress in cancer therapy is to uncover an organizing principle in cancer cell transformations towards greater and greater malignancy. We know that cells become cancerous as a result of complex genetic and epigenetic reprogramming involving complicated regulatory networks leading to their immortality and uncontrolled division. Hundreds of oncotargets have been identified and some therapeutics developed aiming at their inhibition. It is clear that we can't inhibit all oncotargets at once since multiple overlapping toxicities would first kill the patient. Moreover, we cannot possibly inhibit the oncotargets also because cancer cells are plastic and if challenged, they start quiescence programs and "learn" how to survive. Much of our selection of cancer targets and the development of therapies is very *ad hoc* and lacks a consistent logical basis. Based on our preliminary studies we hypothesize that cancer can be characterized by a tendency, which is consistent with a stability criterion for a corresponding thermodynamic function of state. One such trend is to maximize entropy at all levels of the hierarchical organization from DNA to tumor tissue. We have shown is several examples that an analogous criterion may involve a trend towards a Gibbs free energy minimum. In both cases cancer initiation and progression follows a predictive trajectory in a thermodynamic phase space. This is in contrast to normal cells whose main dynamical objective is homeostasis (stability around its defined equilibrium state) and orchestrated functioning in concert with other tissues to serve the organism. Cancer cells do not fulfill these objectives. By contrast, they eliminate a number of cell cycle checkpoints and simplify their program to achieve two main goals: immortality and cell division. Analyzing cancer hallmarks from DNA mutations, to histone methylation, to DNA packaging, to aneuploidy, to cell metabolism (the Warburg effect), to cell morphology, to cell-organization (epithelial to mesenchymal transformation), to (fractal) tumor morphology and even to metastases, one can introduce an organizing principle at all levels of transformations in cancer, which involves a tendency to evolve its thermodynamic state function (entropy increase or Gibbs free energy decrease).

In this chapter we advanced a hypothesis at all levels of biological organization as described above and drawn practical conclusions in terms of both prognostic information for cancer patients and therapeutic interventions that would be aimed at reversing the process in order to reduce entropy resulting in slowing down or even halting the progression of cancer. This involves the critical question of the optimal selection of the molecular therapeutic targets in order to control cancer cell proliferation viewed here as a tendency to a maximum entropy state. While there is an acute need for developing better anti-cancer drugs, the lengthy time and huge costs associated with cancer drug development, together with high failure rates and limited efficacy of targeted drugs necessitate alternative approaches to cancer drug discovery and novel treatment methods. These approaches should not be simply different from the standard of care but should be based on rational hypotheses. In fact, we propose a completely new and ground-breaking paradigm shift from a descriptive to a quantitative measure of cancer based on the application of a physical organizing principle that of entropy maximization or Gibbs free energy minimization as a specific representation of this principle under thermodynamics constraints. In a nutshell, as Erwin Schrödinger famously pondered in his seminal book "What is Life" [4], life is a tendency to reduce entropy of a system, in contrast to inanimate systems, which left to themselves, increase entropy. We hypothesize that cancer, as a pathological, unsustainable state of a living organism is also characterized by entropy increase leading to disorder, disorganization and ultimately death. Reversing this tendency by a variety of therapeutic means including appropriate nutrition, exercise and specifically selected pharmacological agents has a potential of preventing this trend from continuing towards the patient's demise.

Acknowledgments E.A.R. acknowledges funding from CSTS Healthcare, Toronto, Canada. J.A.T. has been supported by funding from the Natural Sciences Engineering Research Council of Canada and the Allard Foundation.

References

1. Kuhn TS, Hawkins D (1963) The structure of scientific revolutions. Am J Phys 31:554–555. doi:10.1119/1.1969660
2. McQuarrie DA (1973) Statistical thermodynamics. Harper & Row, New York
3. Tseng C-Y, Tuszynski J (2015) A unified approach to computational drug discovery. Drug Discov Today 20:1328–1336. doi:10.1016/j.drudis.2015.07.004
4. Schrödinger E (1967) What is life?: the physical aspects of living cell with mind and matter and autobiographical sketches. Cambridge University Press, Cambridge
5. Shannon CE (2001) A mathematical theory of communication. ACM SIGMOBILE Mobile Comput Commun Rev 5:3–55
6. Hanahan D, Weinberg RA (2000) The hallmarks of cancer. Cell 100:57–70
7. Hanahan D, Weinberg RA (2011) Hallmarks of cancer: the next generation. Cell 144:646–674. doi:10.1016/j.cell.2011.02.013
8. Boveri T (1929) The origin of malignant tumors. Lippincott, Williams & Wilkins, Baltimore
9. Holland AJ, Cleveland DW (2009) Boveri revisited: chromosomal instability, aneuploidy and tumorigenesis. Nat Rev Mol Cell Biol 10:478–487. doi:10.1038/nrm2718
10. Stoler DL, Chen N, Basik M, Kahlenberg MS, Rodriguez-Bigas MA, Petrelli NJ, Anderson GR (1999) The onset and extent of genomic instability in sporadic colorectal tumor progression. Proc Natl Acad Sci U S A 96:15121–15126
11. Loeb LA, Springgate CF, Battula N (1974) Errors in DNA replication as a basis of malignant changes. Cancer Res 34:2311–2321
12. Loeb LA, Loeb KR, Anderson JP (2003) Multiple mutations and cancer. Proc Natl Acad Sci U S A 100:776–781. doi:10.1073/pnas.0334858100

13. Nowak MA, Komarova NL, Sengupta A, Jallepalli PV, Shih I-M, Vogelstein B, Lengauer C (2002) The role of chromosomal instability in tumor initiation. Proc Natl Acad Sci U S A 99:16226–16231. doi:10.1073/pnas.202617399

14. Tomasetti C, Vogelstein B (2015) Cancer etiology. Variation in cancer risk among tissues can be explained by the number of stem cell divisions. Science 347:78–81. doi:10.1126/science.1260825

15. Vander Heiden MG, Locasale JW, Swanson KD, Sharfi H, Heffron GJ, Amador-Noguez D, Christofk HR, Wagner G, Rabinowitz JD, Asara JM, Cantley LC (2010) Evidence for an alternative glycolytic pathway in rapidly proliferating cells. Science 329:1492–1499. doi:10.1126/science.1188015

16. Rietman EA, Friesen DE, Hahnfeldt P, Gatenby R, Hlatky L, Tuszynski JA (2013) An integrated multidisciplinary model describing initiation of cancer and the Warburg hypothesis. Theor Biol Med Model 10:39. doi:10.1186/1742-4682-10-39

17. Breitkreutz D, Hlatky L, Rietman E, Tuszynski JA (2012) Molecular signaling network complexity is correlated with cancer patient survivability. Proc Natl Acad Sci U S A 109:9209–9212. doi:10.1073/pnas.1201416109

18. Benzekry S, Tuszynski JA, Rietman EA, Lakka Klement G (2015) Design principles for cancer therapy guided by changes in complexity of protein-protein interaction networks. Biol Direct 10:32. doi:10.1186/s13062-015-0058-5

19. Danø S, Sørensen PG, Hynne F (1999) Sustained oscillations in living cells. Nature 402:320–322. doi:10.1038/46329

20. Voronina S, Sukhomlin T, Johnson PR, Erdemli G, Petersen OH, Tepikin A (2002) Correlation of NADH and Ca2+ signals in mouse pancreatic acinar cells. J Physiol Lond 539:41–52

21. Berridge MJ (2008) Smooth muscle cell calcium activation mechanisms. J Physiol Lond 586:5047–5061. doi:10.1113/jphysiol.2008.160440

22. Vergun O, Votyakova TV, Reynolds IJ (2003) Spontaneous changes in mitochondrial membrane potential in single isolated brain mitochondria. Biophys J 85:3358–3366. doi:10.1016/S0006-3495(03)74755-9

23. Carels N, Tilli T, Tuszynski JA (2015) A computational strategy to select optimized protein targets for drug development toward the control of cancer diseases. PLoS One 10:e0115054. doi:10.1371/journal.pone.0115054

24. Carels N, Tilli TM, Tuszynski JA (2015) Optimization of combination chemotherapy based on the calculation of network entropy for protein-protein interactions in breast cancer cell lines. EPJ Nonlinear Biomed Phys 3:1–18. doi:10.1140/epjnbp/s40366-015-0023-3

25. Porat-Shliom N, Chen Y, Tora M, Shitara A, Masedunskas A, Weigert R (2014) In vivo tissue-wide synchronization of mitochondrial metabolic oscillations. Cell Rep 9:514–521. doi:10.1016/j.celrep.2014.09.022

26. Rietman E, Bloemendal A, Platig J, Tuszynski J, Klement GL (2015) Gibbs free energy of protein-protein interactions reflects tumor stage. bioRxiv. doi:10.1101/022491

27. Greenbaum D, Colangelo C, Williams K, Gerstein M (2003) Comparing protein abundance and mRNA expression levels on a genomic scale. Genome Biol 4:117. doi:10.1186/gb-2003-4-9-117

28. Maier T, Güell M, Serrano L (2009) Correlation of mRNA and protein in complex biological samples. FEBS Lett 583:3966–3973. doi:10.1016/j.febslet.2009.10.036

29. Kim M-S, Pinto SM, Getnet D, Nirujogi RS, Manda SS, Chaerkady R, Madugundu AK, Kelkar DS, Isserlin R, Jain S, Thomas JK, Muthusamy B, Leal-Rojas P, Kumar P, Sahasrabuddhe NA, Balakrishnan L, Advani J, George B, Renuse S, Selvan LDN, Patil AH, Nanjappa V, Radhakrishnan A, Prasad S, Subbannayya T, Raju R, Kumar M, Sreenivasamurthy SK, Marimuthu A, Sathe GJ, Chavan S, Datta KK, Subbannayya Y, Sahu A, Yelamanchi SD, Jayaram S, Rajagopalan P, Sharma J, Murthy KR, Syed N, Goel R, Khan AA, Ahmad S, Dey G, Mudgal K, Chatterjee A, Huang T-C, Zhong J, Wu X, Shaw PG, Freed D, Zahari MS, Mukherjee KK, Shankar S, Mahadevan A, Lam H, Mitchell CJ, Shankar SK, Satishchandra P, Schroeder JT, Sirdeshmukh R, Maitra A, Leach SD, Drake CG, Halushka MK, Prasad TSK,

Hruban RH, Kerr CL, Bader GD, Iacobuzio-Donahue CA, Gowda H, Pandey A (2014) A draft map of the human proteome. Nature 509:575–581. doi:10.1038/nature13302

30. Wilhelm M, Schlegl J, Hahne H, Moghaddas Gholami A, Lieberenz M, Savitski MM, Ziegler E, Butzmann L, Gessulat S, Marx H, Mathieson T, Lemeer S, Schnatbaum K, Reimer U, Wenschuh H, Mollenhauer M, Slotta-Huspenina J, Boese J-H, Bantscheff M, Gerstmair A, Faerber F, Kuster B (2014) Mass-spectrometry-based draft of the human proteome. Nature 509:582–587. doi:10.1038/nature13319

31. Liu R, Li M, Liu Z-P, Wu J, Chen L, Aihara K (2012) Identifying critical transitions and their leading biomolecular networks in complex diseases. Sci Rep 2:813. doi:10.1038/srep00813

32. Berretta R, Moscato P (2010) Cancer biomarker discovery: the entropic hallmark. PLoS One 5:e12262. doi:10.1371/journal.pone.0012262

33. Rietman EA, Platig J, Tuszynski JA, Lakka Klement G (2016) Thermodynamic measures of cancer: Gibbs free energy and entropy of protein-protein interactions. J Biol Phys. doi:10.1007/s10867-016-9410-y

34. Lapointe J, Li C, Higgins JP, van de Rijn M, Bair E, Montgomery K, Ferrari M, Egevad L, Rayford W, Bergerheim U, Ekman P, DeMarzo AM, Tibshirani R, Botstein D, Brown PO, Brooks JD, Pollack JR (2004) Gene expression profiling identifies clinically relevant subtypes of prostate cancer. Proc Natl Acad Sci U S A 101:811–816. doi:10.1073/pnas.0304146101

35. Tomlins SA, Mehra R, Rhodes DR, Cao X, Wang L, Dhanasekaran SM, Kalyana-Sundaram S, Wei JT, Rubin MA, Pienta KJ, Shah RB, Chinnaiyan AM (2007) Integrative molecular concept modeling of prostate cancer progression. Nat Genet 39:41–51. doi:10.1038/ng1935

36. Wurmbach E, Chen Y, Khitrov G, Zhang W, Roayaie S, Schwartz M, Fiel I, Thung S, Mazzaferro V, Bruix J, Bottinger E, Friedman S, Waxman S, Llovet JM (2007) Genome-wide molecular profiles of HCV-induced dysplasia and hepatocellular carcinoma. Hepatology 45:938–947. doi:10.1002/hep.21622

37. Gillies RJ, Raghunand N, Karczmar GS, Bhujwalla ZM (2002) MRI of the tumor microenvironment. J Magn Reson Imaging 16:430–450. doi:10.1002/jmri.10181

38. Gatenby RA, Gillies RJ (2004) Why do cancers have high aerobic glycolysis? Nat Rev Cancer 4:891–899. doi:10.1038/nrc1478

39. Kroemer G, Pouyssegur J (2008) Tumor cell metabolism: cancer's Achilles' heel. Cancer Cell 13:472–482. doi:10.1016/j.ccr.2008.05.005

40. Vander Heiden MG, Cantley LC, Thompson CB (2009) Understanding the Warburg effect: the metabolic requirements of cell proliferation. Science 324:1029–1033. doi:10.1126/science.1160809

41. López-Lázaro M (2010) A new view of carcinogenesis and an alternative approach to cancer therapy. Mol Med 16:144–153. doi:10.2119/molmed.2009.00162

42. Ferrannini E (1988) The theoretical bases of indirect calorimetry: a review. Metab Clin Exp 37:287–301

43. Friesen DE, Baracos VE, Tuszynski JA (2015) Modeling the energetic cost of cancer as a result of altered energy metabolism: implications for cachexia. Theor Biol Med Model 12:17. doi:10.1186/s12976-015-0015-0

44. Johns N, Stephens NA, Fearon KCH (2013) Muscle wasting in cancer. Int J Biochem Cell Biol 45:2215–2229. doi:10.1016/j.biocel.2013.05.032

45. Warburg O (1956) On the origin of cancer cells. Science 123:309–314

46. Davies PC, Demetrius L, Tuszynski JA (2011) Cancer as a dynamical phase transition. Theor Biol Med Model 8:30. doi:10.1186/1742-4682-8-30

47. Zmeskal O, Dzik P, Vesely M (2013) Entropy of fractal systems. Comput Math Appl 66:135–146. doi:10.1016/j.camwa.2013.01.017

48. de Arruda PFF, Gatti M, Facio FN, de Arruda JGF, Moreira RD, Murta LO, de Arruda LF, de Godoy MF (2013) Quantification of fractal dimension and Shannon's entropy in histological diagnosis of prostate cancer. BMC Clin Pathol 13:6. doi:10.1186/1472-6890-13-6

49. Weinan E, Lu J, Yao Y (2012) The landscape of complex networks. arXiv:1204.6376 [physics, q-bio, stat]

50. Van der Toom EE, Verdone JE, Pienta KJ (2016) Disseminated tumor cells and dormancy in prostate cancer metastasis. Curr Opin Biotechnol 40:9–15
51. Dai Y, Wang L, Tang J, Cao P, Luo Z, Sun J, Kiflu A, Sai B, Zhang M, Wang F, Li G (2016) Activation of anaphase-promoting complex by p53 induces a state of dormancy in cancer cells against chemotherapeutic stress. Oncotarget 7:25478–25492
52. Kareva I, Berezovskaya F (2015) Cancer immunoediting: a process driven by metabolic competition as a predator–prey–shared resource type model. J Theor Biol 380:463–472

Printed in the United States
By Bookmasters